Wellbeing in Politics and Policy

Series Editors
Ian Bache
University of Sheffield
Sheffield, UK

Karen Scott
Exeter University (Cornwall Campus)
Penryn, Cornwall, UK

Paul Allin
Imperial College London
London, UK

Wellbeing in Politics and Policy will bring new lenses through which to understand the significance of the dramatic rise of interest in wellbeing as a goal of public policy. While a number of academic disciplines have been influential in both shaping and seeking to explain developments, the Politics discipline has been relatively silent, leaving important theoretical and empirical insights largely absent from debates: insights that have increasing significance as political interest grows. This series will provide a distinctive addition to the field that puts politics and policy at the centre, while embracing interdisciplinary contributions. Contributions will be encouraged from various subfields of the discipline (e.g., political theory, comparative politics, governance and public policy, international relations) and from those located in other disciplines that speak to core political themes (e.g., accountability, gender, inequality, legitimacy and power). The series will seek to explore these themes through policy studies in a range of settings – international, national and local. Comparative studies – either of different policy areas and/or across different settings – will be particularly encouraged. The series will incorporate a wide range of perspectives from critical to problem-solving approaches, drawing on a variety of epistemologies and methodologies. The series welcomes Pivots, edited collections and monographs.

More information about this series at
http://www.palgrave.com/gp/series/15247

Annie Austin

A Universal Declaration of Human Well-being

palgrave
macmillan

Annie Austin
University of Manchester
Manchester, UK

Wellbeing in Politics and Policy
ISBN 978-3-030-27106-0 ISBN 978-3-030-27107-7 (eBook)
https://doi.org/10.1007/978-3-030-27107-7

This Palgrave Pivot imprint is published by the registered company Springer Nature Switzerland AG
The registered company address is: Gewerbestrasse 11, 6330 Cham, Switzerland

For Jeff and Joe

Preface and Acknowledgements

The study documented in this book is based on years of research into well-being, in different contexts and philosophical traditions. It is about the remarkable similarities between human beings, and what human beings think, and have thought, about what makes life good, or meaningful, or worth living. Our common biology entails universal basic needs—food, shelter, clean air and water, and so on. Humans are universally dependent on their environment and on their fellow humans. But this study is not about the universals of human life, but the universals of a *good* human life. Thinking about humanity sometimes starts from the differences between us. This study starts with the idea that, when it comes down to it, people are not so individual and unique as some of us might like to think. The things that make life worth living are strikingly similar across people and peoples. Wildly different philosophies, traditions and cultures have come to the same conclusions. This study explores the common ground that lies beneath the dazzling diversity of humankind.

I am incredibly lucky to benefit from the personal and professional support of a great many people. Thank you to John O'Neill for being a constant source of wisdom and encouragement. Thank you to Ian Bache, Karen Scott and Paul Allin for their guidance throughout this project. The seed of the project was sown during my doctoral research at the Cathie Marsh Institute for Social Research at the University of Manchester—I am indebted to everyone there, and thanks again to John O'Neill and to Nick Shryane for being thoroughly brilliant advisors.

I am grateful to the participants of the ESRC seminar series, *Wellbeing in Politics and Policy* and to my friends and colleagues at the Human Development and Capabilities Association, who have contributed in so many ways to the growth of the ideas in this book. My colleagues at the Centre for Social Ethics and Policy at Manchester have inspired and spurred me on throughout. Most of all, I thank my family, especially Stephen Jeffares, Joseph Austin Jeffares, and Deborah Austin and Allan Austin. Their love and support and critical engagement with this project have kept me going, and are proof positive of my conviction that nothing matters as much as connection with others.

Manchester, UK Annie Austin

Contents

List of Tables

CHAPTER 1

Well-being in Politics and Policy

Abstract What is the ultimate goal of Politics and Policy? This introductory chapter suggests that the best answer to this question is "Well-being": The ultimate goal of politics and policy should be to ensure that citizens are able to live good, flourishing lives. In the twentieth century, politics and policy erroneously inverted its means and ends: Instead of making human well-being its ultimate goal, it focused on economic prosperity, measured by GDP. Resulting policies often treated citizens as mere means to the end of a sound economy. However, in the early twenty-first century, GDP "fetishism" was identified as the fundamental mistake it is, and Politics and Policy were called upon to go "Beyond GDP", and focus directly on human well-being. But what is human well-being? Surely everyone has their own conception of the good? This chapter argues that, given our common biology and common sociality, it would be surprising if there were no universals of human well-being. This study will employ a suite of methods, including documentary analysis of national constitutions, analysis of political "Beyond GDP" programmes, and analysis of the World Values Survey, to identify a universal core of human well-being, as a foundation for people-centred politics and policy.

Keywords Well-being · Flourishing · Beyond GDP · Sociality · Values

A. Austin, *A Universal Declaration of Human Well-being*,
Wellbeing in Politics and Policy,
https://doi.org/10.1007/978-3-030-27107-7_1

What is the ultimate goal of politics and public policy? One answer is that, in an ideal world at least, the ultimate aim of politics and policy is to ensure that citizens are able to live good, flourishing lives. National constitutions and the manifestos of political parties are often a testament to this. To cite just a few examples, the preamble to the US constitution cites the "general welfare" of the people as a core concern,[1] and the constitution of Kenya declares a commitment to "nurturing and protecting the well-being of the individual, the family, communities and the nation."[2] The Manifesto of Spain's largest political party, the *Partido Popular*, states that the person is "the centre, the beginning and the end of all our political action,"[3] while Japan's largest party, the Liberal Democratic Party of Japan, sees "the Public's welfare as our chief imperative."[4]

This political principle of the ultimate value of well-being, however, was seriously compromised during the latter half of the twentieth century by the way in which human welfare was conceptualised and measured. National governments and international institutions tended to equate human welfare with economic welfare, and measured progress and development in terms of macroeconomic indicators like Gross Domestic product (GDP). The "rising tide lifts all boats" approach to economic governance was applied with particular force by international institutions such as the International Monetary Fund and World Bank (for example, through policies of "Structural Adjustment"), often with devastating consequences for human well-being in developing countries.

The main problem with the measurement of human welfare in terms of economic production and consumption alone, and the consequent single-minded focus on macroeconomic policy, is that it subverts the idea that human welfare is of ultimate concern. It amounts to an erroneous inversion of means and ends, often treating citizens as mere means to achieving the end of a sound economy.

[1] Constitution of the United States of America (1789 rev. 1992). Available at https://constituteproject.org/constitution/United_States_of_America_1992.pdf?lang=en (accessed January 2019).

[2] Constitution of Kenya. (2010). Available at https://constituteproject.org/constitution/Kenya_2010.pdf?lang=en (accessed January 2019).

[3] http://www.pp.es/sites/default/files/documentos/estatutos_definitivos.pdf (accessed January 2019).

[4] https://www.jimin.jp/english/about-ldp/history/104257.html (accessed January 2019).

At the beginning of the twenty-first century, however, "GDP fetishism" was identified as the fundamental mistake that it is, largely thanks to the landmark work of Joseph Stiglitz and colleagues (Stiglitz et al. 2009, known as the "Sarkozy Commission"). This represented a breakthrough moment in historic trends of human development, and fired the starting pistol for a new movement whereby national governments and international institutions began to put *people* at the heart of national progress and well-being thinking and policy. At last, it looked as if policy attention had shifted towards people-centred progress that focused on ensuring flourishing lives for people, with a strong economy as just one means of achieving that end. This seemed to be the beginning of a move away from policies grounded in a utilitarian conception of well-being as individual utility, measured at the aggregate level by economic production and consumption, towards a richer conception of the good human life.

Despite some lingering utilitarian tendencies on the part of some national governments (see Chapter 2), the tide had indeed turned. In the wake of the Sarkozy Commission, many national well-being programmes were developed; this has been referred to as the "second wave" of political concern with well-being (Bache and Reardon 2013). Examples include the Bhutanese Gross National Happiness Index, composed of the nine domains of Psychological well-being, Health, Education, Time use, Cultural diversity and resilience, Good governance, Community vitality, Ecological diversity and resilience, and Living standards (Ura et al. 2012), and the Canadian Index of Well-being, constituted by the domains of Community vitality, Democratic engagement, Education, Environment, Healthy populations, Leisure and culture, Living standards and Time use (CIW 2016). In the UK, the Measuring National Well-being programme is designed to "measure what matters" (ONS 2011, p. 2)—that is, what people value. This framework comprises the domains of Health, Relationships, Education and skills, Personal Finance, Where we live, What we do, Personal Well-being, Economy, Governance and Environment (ONS 2011).

These are just three examples of the plethora of national well-being indices developed during the "Beyond GDP" era.[5] There is clear convergence in many aspects of these different frameworks: common to the Canadian, British and Bhutanese lists, for example, are Health, Education, Material standard of living and Social relationships. However, at the same

[5] Of course, GDP remains an important measure of national economic progress; some programmes are framed as "GDP and Beyond." However, second wave initiatives tend to include the Economy as just one aspect of the social setting of well-being, and so go "Beyond GDP" as a proxy for human well-being.

time, important differences remain. Do the Spanish, Japanese and Kenyan governments, for example, have the same conception of what well-being is? This seems unlikely. Societies differ in their political, social and economic structures, and in attitudes and norms around a huge variety of issues. In his classic study of democracies, Lijphart (1999) identified seven "issue dimensions" along which states (democratic or otherwise) vary. These were labelled "Socio-economic," "Religious," "Cultural-ethnic," "Urban-rural," "Regime support" (i.e. popular support for an existing political system), "Foreign policy" and "Post-materialist" (i.e. the balance between what Inglehart (1977) identified as "survival" values, such as material security and stability, and "self-expression" values, such as environmental protection and gender equality). Intersecting variations across all these dimensions result in great diversity in the social-political settings of well-being across the world.

How important are these differences in the context of global challenges such as climate change, poverty and inequality, which require collective action? Differences in "cultural values" are often cited as reasons for conflict and a lack of integration and understanding between people from different countries, and between different communities within the same countries. Indeed, the defence and promotion of "British Values" has featured prominently in British political discourse in recent years, and exclusionary political discourses around "our" values have also found footholds in other countries, notably the Netherlands and the USA.

Diversity in conceptions of what matters most in life raises questions about the most important aspects of human well-being, and whether there are any true universals, or only culture-specific values. The aim of this book is to identify the commonalities that emerge from different theoretical and practical accounts of well-being. I propose that the universal features of the human experience, including our shared embodiment and shared sociality, are grounds for expecting to find commonalities in the basic conceptions of the good that lie beneath the rich diversity of human tradition and culture. The basic needs of human physical survival, such as food and shelter, are obviously universal. However, this study is not about the universals of life, but the universals of a *good* life. Bringing together theoretical and empirical insight about what matters most in life, this study seeks common ground among conceptions of the good across time, tradition, language and culture. The central idea is this: If certain aspects of life are valued consistently across time and tradition, then this suggests that there may be good reason to value those things. The implications for politics and policy at the national and intergovernmental levels are discussed in Part III. Could a Universal Declaration of Human Well-being provide a foundation for national and global governance frameworks aimed at unity, peace and justice?

1.1 Methodology and Methods: Reflective Equilibrium

The analysis will be conducted within the methodology of Reflective Equilibrium (RE), originally introduced by Rawls (1972) in *A Theory of Justice*. In its original form, RE was an approach to justifying ethical beliefs by balancing particular moral judgements with general moral principles. "Narrow" RE involves an iterative balancing process between particular cases and a set of directly related principles, while "Wide" RE broadens the balancing process to include a wider set of theories, including competing moral perspectives, and social and political theories (Rawls 1974).

A further extension of RE is to bring in empirical knowledge. For example, Wolff and de-Shalit (2007) developed "Dynamic Public Reflective Equilibrium" (DPRE), whereby the intuitions and principles of third parties are included in the balancing exercise. In Wolff and de-Shalit's work, members of the British and Israeli publics were asked for their views on the constituents of a good life, and these views were incorporated into the balancing procedure, in order to enhance the legitimacy and relevance of the conclusions. The use of empirical variants of RE is also widespread in the fields of bioethics and medical ethics, where the need to incorporate the practical wisdom of professional practice into ethical reasoning is widely recognised (e.g. De Vries and Van Leeuwen 2010). Martha Nussbaum employs a version of empirical RE, combining philosophical reasoning with "years of cross-cultural discussion" (Nussbaum 2000, p. 76) to arrive at a set of political principles which, she argues, are universally necessary constituents of the political setting of well-being.

In this book, I use empirical RE, balancing theoretical reasoning (Part I) with empirical knowledge (Part II) about the kinds of lives people value. The starting hypothesis is therefore that there is a universal core of human well-being, and that the elements of this universal core are discoverable.[6]

[6]Note that this is not a statistical hypothesis to be accepted or rejected based on statistical tests, but a free-standing statement to be explored qualitatively.

To test this hypothesis from the empirical perspective, my account will draw upon three sources of data: first, a comparative documentary analysis of the political constitutions of countries across the world; second, an examination of "second wave" political initiatives around well-being; and third, an analysis of the World Values Survey (WVS, Inglehart et al. 2014). These sources will be used to identify global patterns in what people believe to be most important in life. To my knowledge, this will be the first attempt to use data from such a broad range of countries and cultures as part of a wide reflective equilibrium on well-being. By bringing together these different sources of knowledge, I hope to identify the elements of a universal core of well-being, as a tool for people-centred politics and policy.

1.1.1 Methods

The documentary analysis of national constitutions will comprise a thematic analysis of a selection of countries in Europe, North America, Latin America, Asia and Africa.[7] The themes will be drawn from the analysis of theoretical approaches to well-being in Part I. The aim of the constitutional analysis is to identify the central principles of conceptions of the good at the political level. Well-being happens (or doesn't happen) in a political setting, and a national constitution describes and sets the parameters of this setting.

Where they are available, examination of second wave well-being initiatives will complement the analysis of political constitutions, again using the themes developed in Part I.

The analysis of the WVS will focus on one particular survey question: "For each of the following, indicate how important it is in your life. Would you say it is Very important, Rather important, Not very important, Not at all important? (Family, Friends, Leisure time, Politics, Work, Religion)."[8] Because it is based on a pre-defined list of domains, this question provides only a very broad view of value priorities, within the constraints of this particular set. However, this is sufficient to tell a story about the general

[7]All constitutions are sourced from the Comparative Constitutions project (Elkins et al. 2010).

[8]This question is appealing because, due to its simplicity, it is likely to have high construct validity across countries and languages—for example, the concept of "family" translates very easily. All WVS questions are subject to extensive validity checks.

nature of mass priorities in different countries, as part of a wider reflective equilibrium. Working back and forth between theory (Part I) and practice (Part II) will begin to reveal commonalities in what people value. If people across time, geography, tradition and culture value the same things, and this matches theoretically-derived principles of the good life, then this is grounds to claim that there is good reason to value those things.

1.1.1.1 Case Selection

It is beyond the scope of this study, and also unnecessary, to analyse each of the 195 countries of the world (UN 2019). Instead, a smaller number of cases will be used. Cases for analysis will be selected through a "Most Different" approach to comparative case study analysis (Meckstroth 1975; Seawright and Gerring 2008). On this approach, it is hypothesised that the state of affairs of interest (in our case, the values and principles that characterise conceptions of the good) remains stable while background conditions vary. Given the aim of this study, to show common ground underlying surface diversity, a "Most Different" approach to case selection is an appropriate strategy. This approach is used across the constitutional analysis and the countries selected for World Values Survey analysis. To achieve the greatest diversity among cases, the following cross-case characteristics are leveraged:

- Geography
  - Cases are selected from different continents, and from different regions within continents. For example, countries from North, East, West and Southern Africa are included.
- Language
  - Linguistic diversity is entailed by geographical diversity.
- Religion
  - Cases are selected to include variation in religion, and in the relationships between religion and the state.
- Political history
  - Cases represent a diversity of political histories, including communism, colonialism, authoritarianism and democracy.

- Culture and tradition
  - Cases are selected based on the extent to which traditional practices are integrated into the political setting of well-being, as articulated in national constitutions.
- Stage of economic development
  - Cases vary in levels of economic development, and include countries that receive financial aid, and donor countries.
- Demographic
  - States of different population sizes are included in the sample, from Qatar with a population of less than 3 million, to China with a population of over 1 billion.

A number of pragmatic considerations were also involved in case selection, including data availability and the author's expertise in different regions.

To summarise, the aim of the empirical part of the study is to analyse a sample of cases that are as diverse as possible, in order to explore commonalities in the underlying values and principles of the good life that exist beneath surface-level diversity. More formally, if people across time, geography and culture value X, Y and Z, then this is evidence that there may be good reason to value X, Y and Z, as human beings.

1.2 Universals of Human Well-being?

Before we begin, it is necessary to pre-empt the most serious objection to a universal approach to human well-being. This objection contains both descriptive and normative challenges. First, the objection goes, given the rich diversity of ways of life, across people and across cultures, the search for universals will be fruitless. From the normative perspective, the proposal of universals of human well-being is suspected of being motivated by colonial aspirations to impose dominant (often "Western") values on others. Existing proposals of universals of human life, such as the Universal Declaration of Human Rights, have been subject to this and similar objections.

1.2.1 The Descriptive Challenge

The descriptive challenge—that universals simply do not exist—rightly points out that every person is a distinct individual with their own way of living based on what they value. It might also contain the insight that every person's conception of the good is developed within a particular social setting, including a particular family, community, society and culture. How could universals possibly emerge from all these layers of variation?

The concept of multiple realizability (Nussbaum 2000, p. 77) provides an answer. The universals of biological survival, such as the need for food and shelter, are multiply realised—for example, corn, wheat, rice and millet can all provide staple carbohydrates, just as wood, brick and stone can all provide shelter. Values are analogous. For example, it might be proposed that "Being a respected member of one's community" is of universal value for human beings. The ways in which respect is earned and shown are undoubtedly different in different cultures, but the underlying value is the same. Similarly, while social interaction is a vital part of a good human life, the institutions that uphold sociality, and the ways in which people interact, clearly vary. But again, the underlying value is the same. While the many ways of life that are found across the world may defy generalisation, commonality can be found at the level of underlying values.

1.2.2 Ethical Naturalism

The case for universal human values is supported by Aristotelian ethical naturalism. On this view, evaluating the human good is no different from evaluating the good of other living things—plants and other animals. As Philippa Foot explained in her ground-breaking work *Natural Goodness*, the roots of a tree can be evaluated as "good" when those roots provide nourishment such that the tree flourishes as one of its kind. A deer that runs swiftly excels in the characteristic way that deer (as a species) typically defend themselves against predators, and so it flourishes in the particular form of life that we call "deer" (Foot 2003, pp. 24–34). The characteristics and functionings of human beings are subject to evaluation in exactly the same way. Human sight and hearing, for example, can be described as "good" or "bad." It is also the case, though, that humans are capable of cooperation and compassion, such that bad sight or bad hearing need not necessarily equate to a failure to flourish as a human. Indeed, sociality, care and cooperation are central constituents of the form of life characteristic of the human animal, and are also subject to normative evaluation.

Just as features of the human physical organism can be evaluated, so can the human will (Foot 2003, p. 24). Compassion, for example, is a virtue that gives people reasons and reason to help those in need. From an ethical naturalist point of view, saying that human compassion and compassionate acts are "good" is no different to saying that well-functioning roots are "good" when it comes to trees. As Foot says, "The concept of a good human life plays the same part in determining the goodness of human characteristics and operations that the concept of flourishing plays in the determination of goodness in plants and animals" (p. 44). Another way of saying all this is that human value is grounded in facts about the nature of human life. This opens up the possibility that there are universal values determined by universal aspects of what it is to be human.[9]

In sum, conceptions of the good are manifested differently in different settings, but all the rich diversity of personal, linguistic and cultural difference stands on common human ground. An ethical naturalist account of human values, along with the multiple realizability thesis, together provide an argument for the possibility of universal human values.

1.2.3 The Normative Challenge

There are two related dimensions of the normative challenge, one philosophical and the other political. First, from a philosophical point of view, it may be objected that an inquiry into what people actually value as the basis for a claim about what is valuable makes a fallacious move from fact to value: All people value X, therefore X is valuable. As we have just seen, however, a response to this worry can be made from ethical naturalism: Objective value is grounded in facts about what it is to be human—about human nature. Finding out facts is therefore a necessary first step to working out value. For those objectors who are unconvinced by ethical naturalism, it should be noted that in any case my goal here is not a strongly normative one. My inquiry will address a descriptive question about a normative issue: What do people *believe* to be important in life? Even if universal value-beliefs emerge, I will make no strong claim about proposed universals being "real" or "objectively true." Instead, I will make the more modest claim

[9]A constraint on ethical naturalism is that it refers to a particular time period, namely the current evolutionary epoch of homo sapiens.

that, if people across the world value X, and this accords with theories of well-being across the ages, then this is evidence that there may be good reason to value X. Throughout the book, I use the term "values" to refer to people's beliefs about value, their "basic convictions about what is and is not important in life" (Allport 1961). These are what Dworkin (1993) calls "Critical Interests."

Second, a political worry is that talk of "values" is usually thinly disguised colonialism, tinged with xenophobia and racism, designed to impose a certain set of values on others and to exclude those with different views. My primary defence against this worry is to introduce "bottom-up" sources of knowledge about what people actually value in their lives—the considered judgements that people from different geographical, political, linguistic and cultural communities across the world make about what is important in life. Triangulating this knowledge with theoretical knowledge about well-being will reveal areas of consensus. This way of doing reflective equilibrium is wide along two dimensions: it involves balancing multiple theoretical perspectives with each other, and with the considered judgements of multiple publics. This reflective equilibrium between theoretical and empirical knowledge aims to capitalise on the strengths of both kinds of knowledge.

The book is organised into three parts. Part I examines Well-being in Theory. It explores the major philosophical approaches to well-being (Chapter 2), and examines examples of "populated" theories of well-being (Chapter 3). Part II focuses on Well-being in Practice, through empirical analysis of real-life conceptions of the good in Europe (Chapter 4), North America (Chapter 5), Latin America (Chapter 6), Asia (Chapter 7) and Africa (Chapter 8). Part III brings together the theoretical and practical to demonstrate that, even in the context of geographical, cultural and linguistic diversity, a set of common priorities and goals of a good human life emerge (Chapter 9).

References

Allport, G. W. (1961). *Pattern and Growth in Personality*. New York: Holt, Rinehart and Winston.

Bache, I., & Reardon, L. (2013). An idea whose time has come? Explaining the rise of well-being in British politics. *Political Studies, 61*(4), 898–914.

CIW. (2016). *How are Canadians Really Doing? The 2016 CIW National Report*. Waterloo, ON: Canadian Index of Wellbeing and University of Waterloo.

De Vries, M., & Van Leeuwen, E. (2010). Reflective equilibrium and empirical data: Third person moral experiences in empirical medical ethics. *Bioethics, 24*(9), 490–498.

Dworkin, R. (1993). *Life's Dominion*. London: HarperCollins.

Elkins, Z., Ginsburg, T., & Melton, J. (2010). *The Comparative Constitutions Project*. https://constituteproject.org/?lang=en.

Foot, P. (2003). *Natural Goodness*. Oxford: Clarendon Press.

Inglehart, R. (1977). *The Silent Revolution: Changing Values and Political Styles Among Western publics*. Princeton: Princeton University Press.

Inglehart, R., Haerpfer, C., Moreno, A., Welzel, C., Kizilova, K., Diez-Medrano, J., et al. (Eds.). (2014). *World Values Survey: Round Six—Country-Pooled Datafile Version*. www.worldvaluessurvey.org/WVSDocumentationWV6.jsp. Madrid: JD Systems Institute.

Lijphart, A. (1999). *Patterns of Democracy: Government Forms and Performance in Thirty-Six Countries*. New Haven: Yale University Press.

Meckstroth, T. W. (1975). I. "Most different systems" and "most similar systems" a study in the logic of comparative inquiry. *Comparative Political Studies, 8*(2), 132–157.

Nussbaum, M. C. (2000). *Women and Human Development: The Capabilities Approach* (Vol. 3). Cambridge: Cambridge University Press.

ONS. (2011). *Measuring What Matters: National Statistician's Reflections on the National Debate on Measuring National Well-Being*. Newport: Office for National Statistics.

Rawls, J. (1972). *A Theory of Justice*. London: Oxford University Press.

Rawls, J. (1974). The independence of moral theory. *Proceedings and Addresses of the American Philosophical Association, 47*, 5–22. In *Collected Papers* (1999) (pp. 286–302).

Seawright, J., & Gerring, J. (2008). Case selection techniques in case study research: A menu of qualitative and quantitative options. *Political Research Quarterly, 61*(2), 294–308.

Stiglitz, J. E., Sen, A., & Fitoussi, J. P. (2009). *Report by the Commission on the Measurement of Economic Performance and Social Progress*. Paris: Commission on the Measurement of Economic Performance and Social Progress.

UN. (2019). *Member States*. https://www.un.org/en/member-states/. Accessed 1 May 2019.

Ura, K., Alkire, S., Zangmo, T., & Wangdi, K. (2012). *A Short Guide to Gross National Happiness Index*. Thimphu: The Centre for Bhutan Studies.

Wolff, J., & de-Shalit, A. (2007). *Disadvantage*. Oxford: Oxford University Press Catalogue.

PART I

Well-being in Theory

Part I begins with an examination of different theories of the good life. First, Chapter 2 identifies candidates for universals of well-being that emerge from a range of foundational ethical theories. Next, Chapter 3 shows the areas of overlap between theoretical approaches that have built upon these foundations to develop substantive accounts of the good. Part I lays the theoretical groundwork for the analysis of Well-being in Practice in Part II.

CHAPTER 2

Theories of Well-being: The Foundations

Abstract This chapter discusses foundational ethical theories that provide diverse answers to Socrates' question of what constitutes a good, flourishing life. Classical utilitarianism employs a hedonistic account of well-being, while classical liberalism and rights-based accounts are grounded in a conception of well-being as individual freedom. Aristotelian approaches typically rest on background theories of well-being as living well in the social-political world. The first three candidates for universals of well-being are therefore Happiness (from Hedonism); Freedom (from Liberalism); and Sociality (from Aristotelianism). The Aristotelian-inspired Capabilities Approach (CA) conceptualises well-being as people's capabilities "to live the lives they value - and have reason to value" Sen (1999). The CA will provide the analytical framework for this study. The aim is to discover what people value, as grounds for proposing that, if people across the world universally value particular aspects of life, then this is evidence that there is good reason to value those aspects of life. This strategy amounts to making a strong claim about the first part of Sen's definition (What people do in fact value), and a more modest claim about the second part (What people have reason to value).

Keywords Flourishing · Well-being · Happiness · Capabilities Approach

A. Austin, *A Universal Declaration of Human Well-being*,
Wellbeing in Politics and Policy,
https://doi.org/10.1007/978-3-030-27107-7_2

Theories of well-being are many and varied. This is unsurprising, given that the question of what it means to live well—to live a good, flourishing, happy life—is an extremely old one. In the western tradition, discussions about the good life first appeared in the writings of the ancient Greeks. In response to Socrates' question of how one should live in order to achieve *Eudaimonia*—the highest human good of a successful, flourishing or well-lived life—different philosophers proposed different definitions of *eudaimonia* (the final end or goal) and different means of achieving it. For example, Epicurus defined *eudaimonia* as a life of pleasure, and advocated retreating from the "rat race" and entering his philosophical commune (the "garden of friends") to achieve it (Bergsma et al. 2008). Meanwhile, in the Nicomachean Ethics (NE) Aristotle defined *eudaimonia* as doing and being well in the social world, through the active exercise of human virtues such as courage, honesty and friendliness (NE 1107b18). For Aristotle, pleasure and enjoyment were merely a fortunate by-product of performing any activity well: well-being consists in living a human life (*being*) and doing it *well.*

Further answers to "the Socratic Question" have continued to emerge throughout the ages. While these are sometimes designed explicitly as theories of well-being, they often function as background theories within larger ethical frameworks. Therefore, the strategy in this chapter will be to examine a selection of moral theories with a view to uncovering the background theories of well-being in which they are grounded. The discussion highlights the philosophical features of these theories, the substantive commonalities and differences between them, and their different implications for politics and policy.

2.1 Hedonism: Utilitarianism and the New Science of Happiness

Classical utilitarianism, as it is found in Bentham (1982/1789) and Mill (1986/1859), is the doctrine that the right thing to do is the act which maximises the good. The classical utilitarians conceived of "the good" as pleasure and the absence of pain, hence Bentham's maxim "The greatest happiness for the greatest number." Classical utilitarianism is grounded in a hedonistic theory of well-being; that is, a conception of the good as the best possible balance of pleasure over pain.

The basic tenets of hedonist and desire-fulfilment variants of utilitarianism continue to play a central role in modern politics and policy. For example, in mainstream economic policy, "Social utility functions" are used to analyse the demand and supply of goods and services, as a guide for economic planning. Herein lies the connection between classical utilitarianism and the GDP fetishism that erroneously inverted the means and ends of human well-being (see Chapter 1). Utility functions are designed to model the combination of commodities that will produce the greatest *satisfaction* in an individual or group. When satisfaction is understood as being obtained through the consumption of goods and services, it is easy to see the utilitarian background theory of well-being at work in the political economy of modern society. It is also easy to see that the "New Science of Happiness," as described and advocated by Layard (2005) and others, and epitomised in the use of survey data on the self-reported happiness and satisfaction of citizens for the purposes of policy planning and evaluation—is grounded in classical utilitarian hedonist thinking (Austin 2015).

Most objections to classical utilitarianism relate to its inadequacy as a normative moral framework, such as the "scapegoating" problem whereby, for the sake of the greater good, a utilitarian must accept the punishment of an innocent individual to placate an angry mob. Another problem with the hedonist conception of well-being is that a pleasant state of consciousness, such as happiness or satisfaction, may result from the fulfilment of preferences or desires that are uninformed, adaptive or in some other way harmful to the individual. This objection from adaptive preferences has been advanced by, among many others, Sen (1999) and Nussbaum (2000), who show how people who are disadvantaged (poor, oppressed, unhealthy, alone, abused) may adapt their preferences, desires and aspirations to fit their straitened circumstances. As such, their happiness or satisfaction is an unreliable indicator of the objective quality of their lives.

In short, its insensitivity to objective facts about people's lives means that Hedonism provides only a partial perspective on human well-being. Nonetheless, the subjective state of Happiness is a plausible candidate universal constituent of well-being.

2.2 Political Liberalism: Resources and Rights

One putative benefit of hedonism (in both its classical and modern forms) is that it is a politically liberal approach to well-being. Epicurus and his philosophical commune aside, mainstream hedonism is neutral about the means to the ultimate end of subjective pleasure. Rather than specifying what is required for happiness, it simply stipulates that happiness is the end, and the means to happiness are to be decided by each person for herself. Advocates of hedonist theories of well-being claim that this makes their approach non-paternalist and democratic (e.g. Diener et al. 1999).

2.2.1 Resourcism

Some theorists take an even stronger position and avoid stipulating any final end at all, instead limiting their analysis to the necessary conditions that any person would require in order to pursue whatever her own particular ends (life plans and goals) may be. This strong liberal strategy is exemplified by John Rawls' work on Justice (e.g. Rawls 1971, 2001). Rawls (2001, pp. 58–59) sets out a list of "primary goods"—a set of basic liberties, opportunities and resources that provide individuals with the means to pursue their life plans, whatever they may be:

1. The basic rights and liberties;
2. Freedom of movement, and free choice among a wide range of occupations;
3. The powers of offices and positions of responsibility;
4. Income and wealth;
5. The social bases of self-respect: the recognition by social institutions that gives citizens a sense of self-worth and the confidence to carry out their plans.

Rawls' list is not designed as a theory of well-being. However, it is possible to infer at least a partial background conception of the good. It is clear that Freedom is the most important human good for Rawls. Other substantive values that emerge are Good Work, Access to Power, Material Resources and Self-respect. While the list of primary goods does not contain a complete theory of well-being, it does presuppose that these things play some part in a good life.

A standard objection to political and economic liberalism and neoliberalism, however, is that by focusing only on the circumstances that enable people to define and pursue their own conception of the good, liberalism is insensitive to the actual quality of lives. It pays too little attention to the real, positive freedoms that people have to achieve valuable outcomes. In a socio-economic system that claims to provide all citizens with the resources they need to live a good life, anything less than a good life becomes the "fault" of the individual. In short, social and economic policy based on liberalism is prone to leaving too little room for consideration of structural issues that can result in unfair inequalities in well-being, and shifting the blame for such failures onto individuals.

2.2.2 *Rights-Based Approaches*

As we have seen, the first item on Rawls' list of primary goods is "the basic rights and liberties." Rights are another route into well-being, especially the "Interest Theory" of rights (e.g. Raz 1986), which defines the function of rights as the protection of the *interests* of the right-holder (i.e. the right-holder's well-being).

Rights-based approaches share a central feature of classical liberalism, in that they do not mandate the things that they protect. The good of Freedom is the foundation of rights-based approaches. However, unlike classical liberalism's focus on negative freedoms, rights-based approaches such as the Universal Declaration of Human Rights advocate positive rights in support of particular substantive goods in the social, economic, cultural, political and civil spheres. For example, the Universal Declaration of Human Rights cites the universal value of goods such as Education (Art.26), Good Work (23), a Standard of Living "adequate to secure basic needs" (25), Family Relationships (16), Rest and Leisure (24), and access to and Participation in political and cultural life (21, 27). Practical rights-based approaches such as the Universal Declaration therefore go some way to answering the question, "Freedom to what?"

2.3 Aristotelian Approaches: Virtues and Capabilities

For Aristotle, Ethics is a practical, rather than a theoretical science. The fields of Virtue Ethics, Communitarianism and Ethical Naturalism (Sect. 1.2) are expressions of Aristotelian ethics, and the Capabilities Approach to well-being borrows many Aristotelian insights.

2.3.1 *Virtue Ethics*

As we saw in the introduction to this chapter, in the Nicomachean Ethics (NE), Aristotle argues that the good life is a question of excelling in the functions and operations that comprise a fully human life. For Aristotle, everything has a function, or a reason for being (a *telos*): for example, the *telos* of a knife is to cut; a good knife is one which cuts well. This extends to living things: every plant and animal has "a proper function" which is distinctive of its species (NE 1175a5–10). For example, a good horse is strong and swift, and a good dog is loyal and obedient. They are "good" in the sense of "good of their kind." Human beings are no exception to this. Aristotle discusses various "spheres of action or feeling" that are defining features of being human, and in which human beings can excel to a greater or lesser extent (NE 1107b18), including Fear and Confidence; Pleasure and Pain; and Social conduct. To be and do well in these spheres requires a person to have particular virtues of character: for example, the virtues in the spheres just mentioned are Courage, Temperance and Friendliness. On this view, living a good life means being a good human. Being a good human means possessing deeply embedded dispositions to think and act in certain ways. It is through the full exercise of distinctly human virtues that a person achieves the human *telos* of *Eudaimonia*—a successful, flourishing human life.

The Aristotelian good life is deeply social. This is evident in his statement that "man is by nature a social being" (NE 1097b10), and in extensive discussions of the necessity of community, friends and family throughout the life-course (e.g. NE 1097b8–10; 1155a3–13). The ability to recognise the right kinds of considerations as reasons for action, given specific circumstances, is not developed through abstract reflection, but through life experience—experience of interacting with others in the social-political setting of one's life (NE 1103a14). Being a good human (living a good human life) can only be achieved in a social setting. This gives rise to the most important candidate for a universal good of human life to emerge from Aristotelian ethics: Good social relationships, or Sociality.

2.3.2 *Communitarianism*

The Aristotelian concern with sociality is found in the political philosophy of Communitarianism, which developed as a response to Rawls' political liberalism. Drawing upon Aristotelian ethics, advocates of Communitarianism assume a social conception of the person, as a being who is the product of her sociality, and who cannot be understood outside of her network of social relationships, including her relationships to the social, economic, political and cultural institutions, and the traditions and norms, that make up her social setting (e.g. MacIntyre 1984). Personal well-being is underpinned by community, and ethical reasoning cannot be undertaken in abstraction from this setting. As Aristotle observed, understanding context is a crucial aspect of practical reasoning, at both the individual and group (political) levels. Practical wisdom (*phronesis*) is partly a case of being able to interpret context, and to incorporate this interpretation into practical reasoning about the good life and the good society. The Aristotelian and communitarian idea of the person as a social being embedded in a social setting is shared by feminist philosophers (e.g. Kittay and Feder 2003), who stress the central value of relationships of care in human life, and argue that interdependence, not independence, is a defining feature of the human social animal.

2.3.3 *The Capabilities Approach*

The final approach to well-being to be considered in this chapter is the Capabilities Approach (CA) (Sen 1980; Nussbaum 2000), which borrows many insights from Aristotle. The CA is not a "theory" of well-being, but an analytical framework for conceptualising and evaluating well-being and social justice. It can be used for the assessment of individual and group well-being, the evaluation of social and political institutions, and the design of policy for social change. The foundational claim of the CA is that well-being is a question of people's real freedom to "lead the kind of lives they value—and have reason to value" (Sen 1999, p. 18).

The CA is broadly liberal in the sense that it grounds well-being in freedom and opportunity. The CA's liberalism, however, differs importantly from classical liberalism. A central claim of the CA is that it is not enough to provide people with resources such as the primary goods, because individuals have different abilities to convert resources into valuable "beings and doings," or "functionings" (Sen 1980). Resources are differentially converted into valuable functionings not only at the individual level, but social and environmental "conversion factors" also play a part. These include features of a person's material environment, and the social and political setting in which her life is embedded. Individuals are in constant interaction with this complex social setting, and it is part of their capability to achieve well-being.

Proponents of the CA argue that the aim of public policy ought to be the expansion of capabilities—the space within which people can develop a conception of the good, and have the opportunity and ability to live in accordance with that conception (Nussbaum 2000). The concept of capability contains a rich conceptualisation of the social-political environment in which every human life is embedded. Therefore, unlike classical liberalism, which sees the role of the state as the minimum required to ensure the protection of negative rights of non-interference, the CA is compatible with a strongly positive role for the state, as the primary actor that shapes the social-political setting.

With the role of politics and policy in mind, Martha Nussbaum (2000, pp. 79–80) proposed ten domains that are so important to a good human life that they deserve to be constitutionally guaranteed by states. We come back to the details of Nussbaum's capabilities in Chapter 3. For now, it is enough to note that Nussbaum gives special importance to the capabilities for Affiliation ("Being able to live with and towards others…Having the social bases of self-respect…") and Practical Reasoning ("Being able to form a conception of the good and to engage in critical reflection about the planning of one's life") because these two "organize and suffuse all the others" (p. 82).

Nussbaum's central domains of capability were developed using the Aristotelian method of identifying the components of "truly human functioning" (p. 74). At the same time, the list is informed by Rawls' liberalism, and represents an extension of the list of primary goods: The idea is that living a good life does not require full functioning in each domain, only that people have the capability (freedom) to reach sufficiency in each domain, such that they are able to form, and live in accordance with, their own conception of the good.

2.3.4 *The CA as an Analytical Framework: Values and Well-being*

A key insight of the Capabilities Approach is Sen's claim that well-being is a matter of people's capabilities to lead the lives "they value - and have reason to value." This claim contains two parts. First, well-being is a question of being able to live in accordance with what one believes to be important. On this view, one's (subjective) beliefs about value constitute one's conception of the good. Second, there must be good (objective) reason to hold these values. This second part of the claim refers to there being some objective grounding of a value-belief that renders its object valuable independently of what anyone might think about it. When objective and subjective reasons behind values align, a person can be said to be in "sound prudential form" (Austin 2018).

As stated in Chapter 1, the aim of this book is to discover commonalities in what people value, as grounds for proposing that, if people across the world universally value particular aspects of life, then this is good evidence that there is good reason to value those aspects of life. This strategy amounts to making a strong claim about the first part of Sen's definition (What people do in fact value), and a more modest claim about the second part (What people have reason to value).

2.4 Chapter Summary

This chapter has discussed classical utilitarianism, which employs a hedonistic account of well-being; classical liberalism and rights-based accounts, whose background theories of well-being centre on individual freedom; and Aristotelian approaches, in which a good life means living well in the social-political world. The first three candidates for universals of well-being are therefore Subjective Well-being (from Hedonism); Freedom (from Liberalism); and Sociality (from Aristotelianism). This chapter has laid the groundwork for our inquiry into universals of human well-being. The next chapter continues the inquiry with a discussion of more populated theories of well-being.

References

Aristotle. (1976). *The Ethics of Aristotle: The Nicomachean Ethics* (J. A. K. Thomson, Trans.). London: Penguin Classics.

Austin, A. (2015). On well-being and public policy: Are we capable of questioning the hegemony of happiness? *Social Indicators Research, 127*(1), 123–138.

Austin, A. (2018). Turning capabilities into functionings: Practical reason as an activation factor. *Journal of Human Development and Capabilities, 19*(1), 24–37.

Bentham, J. (1982/1789). *An Introduction to the Principles of Morals and Legislation*. London: Methuen.

Bergsma, A., Poot, G., & Liefbroer, A. C. (2008). Happiness in the garden of Epicurus. *Journal of Happiness Studies, 9*(3), 397–423.

Diener, E., Suh, E. M., Lucas, R. E., & Smith, H. L. (1999). Subjective well-being: Three decades of progress. *Psychological Bulletin, 125*(2), 276.

Kittay, E. F., & Feder, E. K. (Eds.). (2003). *The Subject of Care: Feminist Perspectives on Dependency*. Lanham: Rowman & Littlefield.

Layard, R. (2005). *Happiness: Lessons from a New Science*. New York: Penguin Press.
MacIntyre, A. (1984). *After Virtue* (2nd ed.). Notre Dame: University of Notre Dame Press.
Mill, J. S. (1986/1859). *On Liberty*. New York: Prometheus Books.
Nussbaum, M. (2000). *Women and Human Development: The Capabilities Approach*. Cambridge: Cambridge University Press.
Rawls, J. (1971). *A Theory of Justice*. Oxford: Oxford University Press.
Rawls, J. (2001). *Justice as Fairness: A Restatement*. Cambridge: Harvard University Press.
Raz, J. (1986). *The Morality of Freedom*. Oxford: Clarendon Press.
Sen, A. (1980). Equality of what? In S. M. McMurrin (Ed.), *The Tanner Lectures on Human Values* (Vol. I, p. 195). Cambridge: Cambridge University Press.
Sen, A. (1999). *Development as Freedom*. Oxford: Oxford University Press.

CHAPTER 3

The Conditions and Constituents of Well-being: Overlapping Values

Abstract The question of what it means to live a good life is an ancient one. During the same historical era as the ancient Greeks were working on Socrates' question of what makes a good life, thinkers in other parts of the world were also asking the same thing; for example, Confucius in China, and the Vedic philosophers in India. The Socratic question has continued to occupy the minds of thinkers throughout the ages, and has become an increasingly important part of modern politics and policy. This chapter shows the areas of overlap among accounts of well-being across the ages. First, the parallels between ancient Greek, Confucian, and Hindu ethical frameworks of the good life are discussed. Next, a selection of modern political philosophies of the good are mined for candidate universals. The chapter shows that thinkers across time, geography, tradition and culture have found reason to value certain aspects of human life. These aspects are Social relationships, Work, Leisure, Education, Health (physical and psychological), Aesthetic experience, and Integrity (also known as "Authentic self-direction"). These more detailed accounts add content to the three basic values identified in Chapter 2: Happiness (from Hedonism); Freedom (from Liberalism); and Sociality (from Aristotelianism).

Keywords Well-being · Integrity · Happiness

A. Austin, *A Universal Declaration of Human Well-being*,
Wellbeing in Politics and Policy,
https://doi.org/10.1007/978-3-030-27107-7_3

As we have seen, the question of what it means to live a good life is an ancient one. During the same historical era as the ancient Greeks were working on the Socratic question of what makes a good life, other thinkers in other parts of the world were also asking the same thing; for example, Confucius in China, and the Vedic and Buddhist philosophers in India. The Socratic question has continued to occupy the minds of thinkers throughout the ages, and has become an increasingly important part of modern politics and policy.

This chapter brings together and shows the areas of overlap among "populated" or substantive accounts of well-being, including both ancient and more recent accounts.

3.1 The Ancients

While the ancient Greeks were developing their ethical philosophies (around 500 BCE), the Chinese thinker Confucius was engaged in a strikingly similar project. In answer to the Socratic question of how a person can achieve *Eudaimonia* (a good, flourishing, well-lived life), Aristotle set out a list of virtues that a person should cultivate and practice: Courage, Temperance, Liberality, Magnificence, Magnanimity, Proper ambition, Patience, Truthfulness, Wit, Friendliness, Modesty and Righteous indignation (Justice) (NE 1107b18–20). Meanwhile, Confucius sought the *dao* (the way to becoming a good person) and also advocated a set of character traits that should be cultivated and put into practice. The Confucian virtues are commonly grouped under the five core values of *jen* (humanity, benevolence); *yi* (good, mutually respectful social relationships, starting with the family and extending outwards); *li* (propriety, temperance, courteous observance of etiquette and rites); *zhi* (nurturing and exercising virtue); and *xin* (truthfulness and sincerity in the practical application of the other virtues) (Cleary 1992; Huang 1997; Yao and Yao 2000).

These accounts reveal areas of consensus about the virtues that enabled a person to live a good life in ancient Greece or China. For both Aristotle and Confucius, a good life is lived by a temperate person who avoids extremes in the important spheres of life, and is benevolent, generous and honest. Both emphasise good interpersonal relationships, and many of the virtues in the lists are relational, in the sense that their subject matter is social interaction (Aristotle's Friendliness and Confucius' Benevolence are examples).

A very similar picture of living well is found in Indian Hindu texts. In this tradition, the virtues of truthfulness, kindness, self-control and respect for others (particularly one's elders) are also highly valued (Sen Sharma 2014). Like Aristotle's virtue ethics, in which the right course of action is whatever a virtuous person would do, it is stated in the Hindu *Apastambadharmasutra* that "One should model one's conduct after the conduct that is unanimously approved by [those] who are well-mannered, aged [i.e. experienced], and self-disciplined, and who are free from greed and deceit" (*Apastambadharmasutra* 1.20.6–8, cited in Hacker 2006). As well as this procedural commonality, the core characteristics of the exemplary virtuous person in the Indian text are familiar from the other ancient frameworks.

Finally, the Greek, Chinese and Indian traditions also have in common their emphasis on the importance of political, social and environmental circumstances in being able to live a good life. Beyond the virtues, Aristotle discusses the importance of a person's external circumstances, including a well-functioning state (e.g. NE 1103b2–4), while a Well-governed state and Peace are part of the Chinese and Indian systems. It seems that a traveller from any one of these three ancient civilisations would have encountered familiar social and moral norms in either of the other regions. The Confucian, Hindu and Aristotelian systems are summarised in Table 3.1.

Table 3.1 Ancient conceptions of the good

Daxue *(Confucian values and virtues)* *(Yao and Yao 2000)*	*Dharma* *(Hindu values and virtues)* *(Sen Sharma 2014)*	*Aristotelian virtues* *(Nicomachean Ethics, 1107b18–20)*
• Nurturing virtue • Good family life, respect for parents • Benevolence (Care for others) • Propriety • Knowing reality • Diligence • Honesty • Independence • Mindfulness • Sincerity • Peace • Successfully (morally) governed state	• Right action in accordance with Dharma • Social order • Non-violence • Truth • Kindness • Respect for elders • Economy • Purity • Forbearance • Self-control • Compassion	• Courage • Temperance • Liberality (Generosity) • Magnificence • Magnanimity • Proper ambition • Patience • Truthfulness • Wit • Friendliness • Modesty • Righteous indignation (Justice)

In these ancient conceptions of the good life, many of the individual virtues relate to living well in relation to one's social group. This implies that Sociality is a necessary condition of well-being: To live well is to exercise other-regarding virtues. Exercising other-regarding virtues requires others. Given the necessary relationality of human life, well-being cannot be understood solely in individual terms.

3.2 Modern Political Theory

Many aspects of these ancient ethical systems have stood the test of time. For example, Tan (2003) defends a Confucian conception of the good life, stressing the social-relational nature of personhood in Confucian ethics, and the emphasis on good relationships with others as the foundation of a good life. An important advocate and practitioner of a modern interpretation of ancient Hindu values and virtues was Mahatma Gandhi, especially with regard to the virtues of non-violence and self-control (see e.g. Parekh 1989). Similarly, numerous philosophers have employed the Aristotelian method to create sets of human goods. As we saw in the last chapter, a prominent example is Martha Nussbaum (2000) and her set of "Central Human Functional Capabilities," which combines Rawlsian liberalism with an Aristotelian approach to identifying the most important domains of life that are worthy of constitutional protection. Other notable theoretical accounts of the good in the Aristotelian and Natural Law traditions include Finnis' "Basic Values"; Chappell's "Values and Virtues," and Gomez-Lobo's "Human goods," all shown in Table 3.2 (additional explanatory notes in square brackets).

There are many commonalities between these accounts. Harmonious **social relationships** appear in some guise in every account, including both close social relationships with family and friends, and the social institutions that uphold dignity and self-respect (e.g. Nussbaum). We saw in the last chapter that Rawls (1972) argued for the primary good of "a free choice among a wide range of occupations"; likewise, Meaningful work is included by Finnis, Gomez-Lobo, and Nussbaum (for the latter, work is part of the capability for Affiliation (b)). The importance of an adequate Education that enables people to use their minds effectively is ubiquitous, as is the value of Play. Chappell's list includes the classical hedonist value of Pleasure and the absence of pain, and Nussbaum includes pleasurable experiences and the avoidance of non-necessary pain as part of the capability for Senses, Imagination and Thought. Psychological and emotional

Table 3.2 Modern conceptions of the good

Basic human goods *Finnis (1980)*	*Central Human Functional Capabilities* *Nussbaum (2000)*
• Life [Survival, Health, Reproduction] • Knowledge [Understanding, Education] • Meaningful work • Play • Aesthetic experience • Sociability [peace and harmony among persons, friendship] • Practical reasonableness (Authentic self-direction) • Harmony with a greater than human source of meaning and value	• Life • Bodily health • Bodily Integrity • Senses, imagination and thought [using one's mind to imagine, think and reason, requiring adequate education] • Emotions • Practical reason [Engaging in critical reflection about the planning of one's life] • Affiliation [Relationships with others, the social bases of self-respect] • Other species [the world of nature] • Control over one's environment [political and material]
Values and virtues *Chappell (1995)*	*Human goods* *Gomez-Lobo (2002)*
• Friendship • Aesthetic value • Pleasure and the absence of pain • Health and inner harmony • Reason, rationality and reasonableness • Truth and knowledge of truth • The natural world • People • Fairness • Achievements	• Life • Family and friendship • Work and play • Experience of beauty • Theoretical knowledge • Integrity

well-being are found in Finnis', Chappell's and Nussbaum's lists: Finnis includes "Inner peace"; Chappell calls it "Inner harmony"; and Nussbaum gives a detailed definition of the capability to have and use the emotions. Fourth, the value of Aesthetic experience appears in each of the modern accounts (e.g. Gomez-Lobo's "Experience of beauty"). This has some connections with the importance given to the Natural environment: Chappell and Nussbaum include (respectively) "The natural environment" and the capability to "live with concern for and in relation to animals, plants and the world of nature" (Other species) as basic or central goods.

In the first instance, then, this selection of accounts, developed through philosophical reasoning, converge on specific spheres of the human good: Social relationships, Work, Education, Play, Health (physical and psychological), Pleasure, Aesthetic experience and the Natural environment.

3.3 Practical Reason and Integrity

An important area of overlap relates to reason, knowledge and truth. Across the modern and ancient accounts we find references to, for example, "knowledge of reality" (a Confucian value) and Chappell's "Truth and knowledge of truth." These are connected to the value of **Integrity**, which in turn is connected to the capability for practical reason.

Integrity is the capability to live in accordance with one's conception of the good; with what one has found reasons and reason to value. Integrity therefore encompasses practical reasoning and practical action.

Turning first to the Practical reasoning aspect of Integrity: Aristotle defines practical reasoning as a person's capacity to "deliberate rightly" about "what is conducive to the good life in general" (NE 1140a26–27). Following Aristotle, Nussbaum (2000, p. 79) defines the capability for Practical reason as "Being able to form a conception of the good and to engage in critical reflection about the planning of one's life."

Good practical reasoning requires different kinds of knowledge and the pursuit of different kinds of truth. First is knowledge gained by the cultivation of a reflective connection to the social setting in which one's life is embedded. This is what Aristotle calls Practical Wisdom (*phronesis*). Practical wisdom is a necessary condition of being able to act well in the social world—good practical reasoning must be outward as well as inward facing. Thoughtful engagement with one's social setting is also a core Confucian value. This evokes communitarian claims about the importance of a person's belonging to a community, tradition and culture, and the central place of this setting in practical reasoning. Practical wisdom is fundamentally relational.

Practical knowledge, however, is necessary but not sufficient for good Practical reasoning. The other part of Practical reasoning is the pursuit of "theoretical knowledge" of the good. For the Greeks, contemplation was of paramount importance (e.g. NE 1138b35–1139a16). The pursuit of theoretical knowledge and truth is captured in Nussbaum's capability for

"Senses, Imagination and Thought," part of which is "Being able to search for the ultimate meaning of life in one's own way" (Nussbaum 2000, p. 79). Finnis includes "Harmony with a greater than human source of meaning and value." Religion is an age-old means of seeking knowledge of the good at a transcendental level. Good practical reasoning draws on both practical and theoretical knowledge.

Combining practical and theoretical knowledge results in what might be termed "wide" practical reasoning: the capability to reflect on one's life within the context of one's multidimensional life-world. These two forms of knowledge are directly connected to two defining features of being human: sociality and rationality. Wide practical reasoning in this sense requires basic needs to be met. Living hand-to-mouth disables the capability to take such a perspective.

The second aspect of Integrity is being able to live in accordance with that which one has found reasons and reason to value. Finnis calls this "Authentic self-direction," and it is captured in the various ways that the ancients advocated sincerity, truth and honesty in the practice of virtue; a faithfulness to the good. It is interesting to note that the central Hindu value of *Dharma* can be understood as "conformity with the truth of things" (Chakraborty 2006, p. 91).

Just as the practical reasoning aspect of Integrity is fundamentally relational, so is the practical action aspect. The social settings in which human lives are embedded both inform what people value, and enable or disable them in striving to live in accordance with their conceptions of the good. In everyday language, living with Integrity is sometimes called "being true to oneself." On the relational view of Integrity described here, "being true to oneself" means being true to oneself as a social-relational being who shares identities, interests and ends with others. The relational view of Integrity therefore entails a social conception of the person, whose sociality grounds practical reason and action.

In the wider philosophical literature, Integrity is treated by some (e.g. Dworkin 1993) as the most important value of all. The relational view of Integrity departs from the individualistic conception defended by Kantian-inspired philosophers such as Dworkin, and fits much more naturally with Aristotelian ethics. In addition to the values identified previously, then, and recognising its fundamental relationality, we add the new value of **Integrity**.

3.4 Chapter Summary

This chapter has shown areas of convergence among a selection of theory-based accounts of well-being. First, the parallels between ancient Greek, Confucian and Hindu ethical frameworks of the good life and the good society were discussed. Next, we considered a selection of modern conceptions of the good, all developed through philosophical reasoning. While there is undoubtedly mutual influence between some of the theories considered, it is indisputable that thinkers across time, geography, tradition and culture have found reason to value certain aspects of human life. Those to emerge so far are Social relationships, Work, Leisure, Education, Health (physical and psychological), Aesthetic experience and Integrity. These more detailed accounts have added content to the three basic values identified in Chapter 2: Happiness (from Hedonism); Freedom (from Liberalism); and Sociality (from Aristotelianism). This theory-based set of values provides the foundation of an analysis of well-being in practice (Part II).

References

Chakraborty, D. (2006). Is an Indian ethics of virtue possible? *Journal of Human Values, 12*(1), 91–98.

Chappell, T. (Ed.). (2006). *Values and Virtues: Aristotelianism in Contemporary Ethics*. Oxford: Oxford University Press on Demand.

Cleary, T. (1992). Introduction. In T. Cleary (Trans.), *The Essential Confucius* (pp. 1–11). New York: HarperCollins.

Dworkin, R. (1993). *Life's Dominion: An Argument About Abortion, Euthanasia, and Individual Freedom*. London: HarperCollins.

Goldie, P. (2007). Dramatic irony, narrative, and the external perspective. *Royal Institute of Philosophy Supplements, 60*, 69–84.

Gomez-Lobo, A. (2002). *Morality and the Human Goods: An Introduction to Natural Law Ethics*. Washington, DC: Georgetown University Press.

Hacker, P. (2006). Dharma in Hinduism. *Journal of Indian Philosophy, 34*(5), 479–496.

Huang, C. (Ed.). (1997). *The analects of Confucius*. Oxford University Press on Demand.

Nussbaum, M. C. (2000). *Women and Human Development: The Capabilities Approach*. Cambridge: Cambridge University Press.

Parekh, B. C. (1989). *Gandhi's Political Philosophy: A Critical Examination*. London: Palgrave Macmillan.

Sharma, D. S. (2014). Hindu values. *Asian Values: Encounter with Diversity*, 106.

Tan, S. H. (2003). *Confucian Democracy: A Deweyan Reconstruction*. Albany: SUNY Press.
Yao, H. C., & Yao, X. (2000). *An introduction to Confucianism*. Cambridge University Press.

PART I

Summary of Part I: Well-being in Theory

Part I has examined theoretical and philosophical accounts of well-being, with the aim of identifying commonalities among theories developed at different times and in different places and traditions. The ancient, classical and modern accounts of well-being considered here have yielded the following set of candidate universals of human well-being:

- Sociality (Good social relationships, including family, friendship and the formal institutions of sociality)
- Freedom
- Education
- Meaningful work
- Leisure, play
- Material security
- Health (physical and mental)
- Pleasure (subjective well-being, happiness, emotional well-being)
- Connection with the natural environment
- Aesthetic experience
- Integrity (Harmony between practical reasoning and practical action).

The neo-Aristotelian Capabilities Approach provides the analytical framework of this book. In accordance with the conception of well-being as people's capability to live the lives "they value—and have reason to value," my objective will be to discover what is valued, as a means to identifying what there may be good reason to value. Part I has initiated the inquiry with Well-being in Theory; Part II continues with an analysis of Well-being in Practice.

PART II

Well-being in Practice

The aim of Part II is to identify the core values and principles of social and political conceptions of the good across the world, and to highlight areas of consensus between them. To meet this aim, each part begins with an overview of the political philosophies found in those regions, including "Western" liberalism, Latin American *Buen vivir*, African *Ubuntu*, and Hindu, Confucian and Arabic conceptions of the good life. Then, for each region, three main sources of information are analysed. First, a documentary analysis of national constitutions[1] and other important political and legal instruments shows the underlying principles of the political settings of well-being in each place; second, where they exist, "second wave" well-being initiatives are examined; and third, insights from the World Values Survey show the mass priorities of citizens across the world. Connections between the practicalities of well-being and the theories of well-being discussed in Part I are explored.

At the outset, it is important to draw attention to three influential examples of frameworks relevant to well-being in politics and policy at the national and intergovernmental levels.

The first is the International Bill of Human Rights (IBHR), comprising the Universal Declaration of Human Rights (1948), the International Covenant on Economic, Social and Cultural Rights (1966), the

[1] All constitutions are sourced from the Comparative Constitutions Project (Elkins et al. 2010).

International Covenant on Civil and Political Rights (1966), plus two optional protocols on the latter. Together, these affirm a set of civil, political, economic, social and cultural rights, designed to apply to every human being in every country of the world. The IBHR is an important part of the political and legal settings of well-being across the world.

The second important intergovernmental framework is the Organisation for Economic Cooperation and Development (OECD) Better Life Initiatve, designed to measure social progress among member states. Within this framework, a good life is constituted by doing and being well in the domains of Health, Work-life balance, Education and Skills, Social connections, Civic engagement and governance, Environmental quality, Personal security, Subjective well-being, Income and wealth, Jobs and earnings, plus the "resources for future well-being" of natural, economic, human and social capital. (OECD 2013). This framework was at the forefront of what Bache and Reardon (2013) have called the "second wave" of political concern with well-being, and has been an important influence on national initiatives.

Third, the United Nations' Sustainable Development Goals (SDGs, UN 2015) set out an aspirational vision for the well-being of global society, including individual and household-level considerations such as Health, Education and Income, structural considerations around Just Institutions, and environmental considerations relating to the natural world. The 17 Goals, organised around the three dimensions of economic, social and environmental sustainable development, are a rights-based statement of the good life, whereby economic, social and environmental progress are pursued in an integrated, holistic way. The SDGs were designed as a guide for policy and action in nation states and intergovernmental organisations, and so form part of the political backdrop of well-being across the world.

The following chapters examine conceptions of the good at the political levels in Europe (Chapter 4), North America (Chapter 5), Latin America (Chapter 6), Asia (Chapter 7) and Africa (Chapter 8).

References

Bache, I., & Reardon, L. (2013). An idea whose time has come? Explaining the rise of well-being in British politics. *Political Studies, 61*(4), 898–914.

Elkins, Z., Ginsburg, T., & Melton, J. (2010). *The Comparative Constitutions Project.* https://constituteproject.org/?lang=en. Accessed September–December 2018.

OECD (2013). *Better Life Initiative: Measuring Well-being and Progress.* Paris: OECD.

UN (2015). *Transforming Our World, the 2030 Agenda for Sustainable Development.* New York: United Nations General Assembly Resolution A/RES/70/1, 21 October 2015. https://sustainabledevelopment.un.org/post2015/transformingourworld. Accessed January 2019.

CHAPTER 4

Well-being in Europe

Abstract Well-being happens, or doesn't happen, in a social-political setting. This chapter identifies the main principles and priorities of political settings of well-being in Europe. After a discussion of the dominant political theories found in this region, the central principles of the European Union Constitutional Treaty and Convention on Human Rights are identified. Next, an examination of a selection of country constitutions, along with "Beyond GDP" national well-being initiatives, demonstrates the core values of political conceptions of the good across Northern, Southern, Western and Central-Eastern Europe. Finally, evidence from the World Values Survey reveals the mass priorities of a selection of countries across these different regions. The features of European political conceptions of the good can be described as broadly liberal, with a particular emphasis on the social conditions of well-being.

Keywords Well-being · Europe · "Beyond GDP" · Values

This chapter presents evidence from Europe. After a discussion of the dominant political theories found in this region, the central principles of the European Union Constitutional Treaty and Convention on Human Rights are identified. Next, an examination of a selection of country constitutions, along with "Beyond GDP" national well-being initiatives, shows the core

A. Austin, *A Universal Declaration of Human Well-being*,
Wellbeing in Politics and Policy,
https://doi.org/10.1007/978-3-030-27107-7_4

themes of political conceptions of the good across Northern, Southern, Western and Central-Eastern Europe. Finally, evidence from the World Values Survey reveals the mass priorities of a selection of countries across these different regions. The objective of this chapter is to provide a broad view of the main values operant at the political and population levels in Europe.

4.1 Theories of Well-being

The historical period known as the Enlightenment in Europe was characterised by a prioritisation of the individual and individual rights. Thinkers such as Kant, Locke and Rousseau developed a liberal account of the person, and of the relationship between citizen and state, based on the foundational value of individual freedom. One aim of this liberalism was to free individuals from the arbitrary power of monarchs, the Church, and the bonds of traditional social roles and hierarchies. This historical period is the source of political liberalism as it is found in modern Europe.

Political liberalism is not without its critics. Critics argue that the individualism inherent in theoretical liberalism has been taken too far in practice, leading ultimately to a collapse in the social conditions of well-being. As we saw in Chapter 2, philosophers in the communitarian and feminist ethical traditions have been at the forefront of this critique in modern political theory. Despite these critiques, political liberalism remains a dominant force in Europe.

4.2 Political Settings of Well-being in Europe

4.2.1 The European Union (EU)

The founding treaty of the EU, the Treaty of Rome (1957),[1] states that an important task of the EU is "the raising of the standard of living and quality of life" of its peoples (Art.2). The Treaty on European Union (2012)[2] expands on this, opening with a statement that the Union is founded on the shared values of "respect for human dignity, freedom, democracy, equality, the rule of law, and respect for human rights" (Art.2), in order to "promote

[1] https://eur-lex.europa.eu/legal-content/EN/TXT/HTML/?uri=LEGISSUM:xy0023&from=EN (accessed May 2019).

[2] https://eur-lex.europa.eu/eli/treaty/teu_2012/art_2/oj (accessed February 2019).

peace and the well-being of its peoples" (Art.3.1). Alongside these treaties, the European Convention on Human Rights, based on the International Bill of Human Rights, emphasises individual liberties, rights and duties. These values, focused on individual rights and the conditions for human freedom, are firmly rooted in the liberal enlightenment tradition.

The EU was at the forefront of the "Second wave," with its "Beyond GDP: Measuring Progress, True Wealth and the Well-being of Nations" initiative (EU 2007). This programme aims to improve indicators of progress by complementing economic measures with indicators of environmental protection, and social indicators relating to "Quality of life and well-being" (EC 2009, pp. 4–7), and to support EU bodies and member states in harnessing this information in policy decision making.

While the EU aims to provide a common European identity, each member state has its own priorities and national identity, and different regions have different characteristics. Below we consider the regions of Northern, Southern, Eastern/Central and Western Europe. Taking these regions as single entities clearly smooths over many important differences between individual countries, just as taking an individual country as a whole smooths over important within-country differences. The choice to take a broad regional approach is consistent with the goal of focusing on common ground (see Sect. 1.1 on Case Selection).

4.2.2 *Nordic Conceptions of the Good Life*

The constitutions of the five Nordic countries (Denmark, Finland, Iceland, Norway and Sweden) all centre on protection of the social, economic, cultural, political and civil rights and liberties found in the IBHR, and on the institutions of liberal democratic government. There is little mention of other national priorities beyond the internationally recognised rights. Exceptions to this include the Norwegian constitution's opening statement that "Our values will remain our Christian and humanistic heritage. This Constitution shall ensure democracy, a state based on the rule of law and human rights" (Art.1). Another exception, also from the Norwegian constitution, is the guarantee of state protection for the right of the indigenous Sami people "to preserve and develop its language, culture and way of life" (Art.108). Overall, these constitutions draw upon international human rights instruments to set out a fundamentally liberal vision of the good society, as one that underpins the basic conditions for citizens to pursue their life plans.

This political liberalism is characteristic of the intergovernmental Nordic Council of Ministers. Within the liberal context, however, their regular State of the Nordic Region report emphasises specific domains of life including Employment, Education, Digitalisation, Health and Welfare, and Culture and the Arts. For example, in the sphere of health and welfare, the report focuses on both physical and mental health, and economic vulnerability and poverty (State of the Nordic Region 2018, Chapter 13). The domain of Culture and the Arts includes the protection of the "historical, cultural and linguistic heritage" of the region (p. 184), and cultural activities relating to cinemas, libraries and museums (Chapter 14).

The Nordic Welfare Watch, a research programme commissioned by the Council, created an index of well-being from a specifically Nordic perspective (Nyman et al. 2016), comprised by nine domains:

1. Health
2. Educational skills
3. Employment
4. Work-life balance
5. Income and earnings
6. Housing
7. Social networks, social support and participation
8. Personal security
9. Subjective well-being.

As we will see, the inclusion of a plurality of domains of objective well-being, plus subjective well-being, is standard practice in "second wave" well-being initiatives, and the influence of the OECD (2013) Better Life Programme can be seen. However, compared to other well-being indices, it is notable that the Nordic version includes work-life balance as a specific and separate constituent, a value in its own right. This consideration moderates the traditional economic measures of employment and income. A related phenomenon in the Nordic region is the so-called Co-living movement, which advocates the development of collective living communities, designed to maximise social interaction, reciprocity and cooperation. The co-living movement (also found in other European countries including the UK and the Netherlands), is a clear manifestation of communitarian values, and is often cited as a reaction to "liberal individualism."

Overall, Nordic political conceptions of the good can be characterised as strongly liberal: the central principle is Liberty, to be protected by rights. This is somewhat moderated by second wave initiatives that aim to promote living well in specific domains, and, in practice, by social policies designed to improve the conditions of well-being: a well-known example includes policies around equitable childcare in Denmark (Randall 2000).

4.2.3 Well-being in Western Europe

The preamble of the French constitution (1958, rev. 2008) declares the nation's commitment to being a republic founded on the classic revolutionary principles of Liberty, Equality and Fraternity. It contains the statement, originally from the 1789 Declaration of Rights, that the aim of all political institutions is the protection of the "natural rights" of "Liberty, Property, Safety and Resistance to Oppression" (XVII.2). For the modern era, the constitution adds the social, economic, political, cultural and civil rights of the IBHR, including rights and duties relating to employment and education, and "the guarantee to all…[of] protection for health, material security, rest and leisure." It also contains a separate Charter for the Environment, which states that the natural environment is "the common heritage of all human beings"; and that "The future and very existence of mankind are inextricably linked with its natural environment." These, and other statements, are the source of a set of environmental rights and duties.

The constitution of the Netherlands (1815, rev. 2008) is similarly rights-based, opening with a Chapter on Fundamental Rights, including the full range of economic, social, cultural, political and civil rights of the IBHR. Special protections are guaranteed for Employment (Art.19); Material living standards and social assistance (Art.20); Health, Housing, and Social and cultural development and leisure activities (Art.22); and the Natural environment (Art.21). Education is "the constant concern of the government" (Art.23).

Overall, their basis in rights makes the constitutions of these countries politically liberal, while the wording of specific rights gives some indication of particular political priorities. For example, the French constitution contains special considerations in relation to the Natural Environment. As the birth-place of the Enlightenment, and the centre of the horrors of twentieth century wars, it is unsurprising that Western European political regimes are underpinned by rights-based constitutions.

4.3 Second Wave Well-being

Many western European nations have embraced the global Well-being agenda at the highest levels of politics and policy, with national indices of well-being developed in several countries, including the UK ("Measuring What Matters"), France (INSEE 2018) and Germany ("What Matters to us"). Germany's 2013 Coalition Agreement stated that "We wish to align our policies more closely with the values and hopes of German citizens and we will therefore conduct a dialogue with them in order to gain an understanding of their views on wellbeing issues" (German Bundestag 2013). Similarly, the UK statistical authority led "a national debate asking 'What matters to you?'" (ONS 2011). Table 4.1 shows the well-being indices resulting from these consultation processes.

Table 4.1 Indices of national well-being: UK, France, Germany

UK	*France*	*Germany*
• Personal well-being (subjective well-being) • Relationships • Health • Where we live (accommodation, crime, security, access to natural environment, services, community) • What we do (employment, leisure time, cultural participation, volunteering) • Personal finance • Economy • Education and skills • Governance (voter turnout, trust in government) • Natural environment	• General satisfaction with life • Social relationships • Health • Housing • Education • Insecurity • Justice • Civic life • Private activities	• Healthy throughout life • Good work and equitable participation • Equal educational opportunities for all • Having time for work and family • A secure income • Living a life in security and freedom • At home in urban and rural areas • Standing together in family and society • Strengthening the economy, investing in the future • Preserving nature, protecting the environment • Living freely and equal before the law • Acting with global responsibility and securing peace

Table 4.1 shows that the domains shared across all three indices are: Health; Education; Social relationships; Housing; Economic security; Work; and Leisure. Other domains include Subjective Well-being, the Natural Environment, and aspects of civic life. Each of these national frameworks has embraced the main domains identified in the OECD Better Life programme.

4.3.1 Well-being in Southern Europe

The countries of "Southern Europe"—Spain, Portugal, Italy and Greece—are often characterised as some of the most traditional societies in Europe, with stronger emphases on family and religion, and more socially conservative attitudes than other countries (e.g. Ferrera 1996). The modern history of these countries is one of transition to democracy, and the shared past of authoritarianism is often cited as the basis of social, economic and cultural similarities between them.

Another common characteristic of the modern, post-autocratic Southern European republics is the adoption of the International Bill of Human Rights (IBHR) as the foundation of their constitutions. The preamble of the Portuguese constitution refers to "the fundamental rights and freedoms" of the people, and Article 1 states that the republic shall be "based on the dignity of the human person." Similarly, the preamble to the Spanish constitution states that the nation will aim to "establish justice, liberty, and security, ...[and] ensure a dignified quality of life for all."

The constitutions of Spain, Portugal, Italy and Greece all incorporate the civil, political, economic, social and cultural rights of the IBHR, with additions relevant to specific aspects of each country's circumstances. For example, the Spanish constitution includes explicit reference to the protection of minority languages as part of Spain's cultural heritage (Art.3.3).

In Italy, as part of the political imperative to "go beyond GDP," the National Statistical Authority produces an annual report entitled "Equitable and Sustainable Well-being in Italy" (Istat 2018), which analyses national well-being in the domains of Health, Education and Training, Employment and Work-Life Balance, Economic Well-being, Social Relationships, Politics and institutions, Security, Subjective well-being, Landscape and Cultural Heritage, and Natural Environment. The Italian approach is representative of the political conceptions of well-being in the other countries of Southern Europe, which can be summarised as a broadly rights-based approach, with a focus on the OECD domains, plus special attention to cultural and linguistic heritage.

4.3.2 Well-being in Central and Eastern Europe

The late twentieth-century collapse of communism in Central and Eastern Europe led to a transitional period in the post-communist states. Some of these states, such as Poland, Estonia, Slovenia, and many others, became members of the EU during the early 2000s. As in Southern Europe, the history of authoritarianism and oppression in this region plays an important part in the political conceptions of well-being in the modern republics. For example, the preambles of the constitutions of Slovenia,[3] Poland[4] and Estonia[5] all include references to the liberal values of freedom and rights, and each of these constitutions incorporates the full range of civil, political, cultural, social and economic rights of the IBHR.

Despite their common foundation in individual freedoms and rights, the constitutions of these countries express particular national characteristics and values. For example, the preamble of the Polish constitution includes the idea that Polish citizens are "Beholden to our ancestors" and "Obliged to bequeath to future generations all that is valuable from our over one thousand years' heritage," plus the invocation of international cooperation for "the good of the human family." These statements represent an explicit claim to a particularly Polish national identity with its own historical and cultural heritage. At the same time it situates the nation within a much wider story of humanity that stretches back into history and forward to the future. As we will see later, the idea that individual well-being relates to being part of a bigger story is a common value elsewhere in the world.

4.4 Mass Priorities in Europe

So far, we have examined political conceptions of the good, as expressed in national constitutions and second wave well-being initiatives. Table 4.2

[3]Constitution of Slovenia (1991, rev. 2016). https://constituteproject.org/constitution/Slovenia_2016.pdf?lang=en (accessed December 2018)

[4]Constitution of Poland (1997, rev. 2009). https://constituteproject.org/constitution/Poland_2009.pdf?lang=en (accessed December 2018).

[5]Constitution of Estonia (1992, rev. 2015). https://constituteproject.org/constitution/Estonia_2015.pdf?lang=en (accessed December 2018).

Table 4.2 Value priorities in a selection of European Countries (% "Very important")

Germany		*Slovenia*		*Spain*		*Sweden*	
Family	77.6	Family	88.7	Family	91.1	Family	89.2
Friends	50.9	Friends	44.2	Work	62.4	Friends	67.8
Work	39.4	Work	41.3	Friends	52.4	Leisure time	53.6
Leisure time	31.6	Leisure time	41.2	Leisure time	44.8	Work	50.3
Religion	13.1	Religion	11.2	Religion	10.7	Politics	17.3
Politics	10.1	Politics	2.0	Politics	5.9	Religion	7.9

Source World Values Survey Wave 6

shows data from the World Values Survey (Inglehart et al. 2014) for a selection of countries across the Western, Eastern-Central, Southern and Northern regions of Europe. It shows the proportion of the population in each country that rated as "Very Important" the values of Family, Friends, Work, Leisure time, Religion and Politics. The values are listed in order of importance for each country.

Table 4.2 shows that Family, Friends and Work are most likely to be rated as "Very important" in these countries, with the exception of Sweden, where Leisure time replaces work in the top three. Without exception, Family is most important, and Religion and Politics are least important. This suggests that, in each of these different countries, close social relationships are at the heart of conceptions of the good. These are only 4 of 28 member states of the EU; however, it seems that, at least with regard to the importance of close social connections, political and popular conceptions of the good in these European countries are aligned.

4.5 Chapter Summary: The "European Model"?

The conception of the good described by the EU treaties and individual country constitutions can be summarised as fundamentally liberal: the goal is to ensure that background conditions are sound, such that citizens can live freely, in accordance with their own conceptions of the good. The rights-based conceptions of the good life found in the regional treaties and individual country constitutions are strongly influenced by the International Bill of Human Rights, which itself was motivated by modern European history. The development of "Beyond GDP" national well-being initiatives has been guided by the substantive values of the OECD "Better Life" framework (see Introduction to Part II), and these play out in policy settings grounded in liberal values.

However, political liberalism as it is manifested in Europe is not based solely on negative rights of non-interference. European countries are characterised by relatively high levels of taxation and large public sectors, including higher than OECD—average welfare spending (OECD 2019). There are many examples of the promotion of positive freedoms; a particularly notable case of policy-led social change is family policy in the Nordic countries, which have become world leaders in gender equality (Thévenon 2011). The pro-active role of the state means that the modern European model is not bare political liberalism. Instead, it exemplifies the "social market economy" advocated in the EU Lisbon Treaty (Art.3.III)—a brand of liberalism with a particularly strong emphasis on the social conditions of well-being. The social market economy is often defined as distinctly "European," in contrast to "American-style" capitalism based on a stronger form of political and economic liberalism.

References

EU. (2007). *Beyond GDP—Measuring Progress, True Wealth and the Well-Being of Nations*. Brussels. https://ec.europa.eu/jrc/en/printpdf/136879. Accessed March 2019.

EC. (2009). *Communication from the Commission to the Council and the European Parliament—GDP and Beyond: Measuring Progress in a Changing World*. Brussels: European Commission. Available at http://eur-lex.europa.eu/Notice.do?checktexts=checkbox&val=499855. Accessed February 2019.

Ferrera, M. (1996). The 'Southern model' of welfare in social Europe. *Journal of European Social Policy, 6*(1), 17–37.

German Bundestag. (2013). *Government Report on Wellbeing in Germany*. Berlin: Federal Press Office. https://www.gut-leben-in-deutschland.de/SharedDocs/Downloads/EN/LB/Government-Report-on-Wellbeing-in-Germany.pdf. Accessed January 2019.

Inglehart, R., Haerpfer, C., Moreno, A., Welzel, C., Kizilova, K., Diez-Medrano, J., et al. (Eds.). (2014). *World Values Survey: Round Six—Country-Pooled Datafile Version*. http://www.worldvaluessurvey.org/WVSDocumentationWV6.jsp. Madrid: JD Systems Institute.

INSEE. (2018). *France, Social Portrait* (2018 ed.). Paris: Institut national de la statistique et des études économiques. https://www.insee.fr/en/statistiques/3646243. Accessed January 2019.

ISTAT. (2018). *Equitable and Sustainable Well-Being in Italy*. Rome: Instituto Nazionale di Statistica. https://www.istat.it/en/well-being-and-sustainability/the-measurement-of-well-being/bes-report. Accessed 18 February 2019.

Nyman, H., Jónsdóttir, S., Blöndal, L., Etwil, P., Helgeson, T., Rønning, E., et al. (2016). *A Nordic Welfare Indicator System (NOVI)—Report for the Nordic Council of Ministers*. Reykjavík, Iceland: Ministry of Welfare.

OECD. (2013). *How's Life? 2013: Measuring Well-Being*. Paris: OECD. http://dx.doi.org/10.1787/9789264201392-en. Accessed 4 December 2018.

OECD. (2019). *Social Spending (Indicator)*. https://doi.org/10.1787/7497563b-en. Accessed 10 March 2019.

ONS. (2011). *Measuring What Matters: National Statistician's Reflections on the National Debate on Measuring National Well-Being*. Newport: Office for National Statistics.

Randall, V. (2000). Childcare policy in the European states: Limits to convergence. *Journal of European Public Policy, 7*(3), 346–368.

State of the Nordic Region. (2018). Nordic Council of Ministers. https://www.nordregio.org/publications/state-of-the-nordic-region-2018/. Accessed January 2019.

Thévenon, O. (2011). Family policies in OECD countries: A comparative analysis. *Population and Development Review, 37*(1), 57–87.

CHAPTER 5

Well-being in North America

Abstract This chapter provides a broad view of the main values operant at the political and population levels in North America: the USA and Canada. First, the theory of Political Liberalism and its modern North American interpretation is discussed. Next, the central principles of important political and legal instruments are identified, and "second-wave" well-being initiatives are examined. Finally, evidence from the World Values Survey reveals mass priorities in this region. Political liberalism provides the basis of political conceptions of the good in North America, with individual freedom as the defining principle. This liberalism is manifested differently in the USA and Canada, with more policy focus on social and economic rights in Canada. Despite worries about the individualism inherent in classical liberalism, findings suggest that, in practice, liberalism does not necessarily entail the devaluation of sociality; social relationships are a mass priority in both countries. Common priorities emerging from second-wave initiatives include Material living standards, Work, Education, Health, and Communities and families, and the World Values Survey shows that family relationships are a top priority.

Keywords Values · North America · Liberalism · Well-being

A. Austin, *A Universal Declaration of Human Well-being*,
Wellbeing in Politics and Policy,
https://doi.org/10.1007/978-3-030-27107-7_5

This chapter gives a broad view of the main values operant at the political and population levels in North America: the USA and Canada. First, the theory of Political Liberalism, and its modern North American interpretation is discussed. Next, the central principles of important political and legal instruments are identified, and "second wave" well-being initiatives are examined. Finally, evidence from the World Values Survey reveals mass priorities in this region.

5.1 North American Liberalism

As we saw in Chapter 2, the central value of classical Liberalism, as it is found in the work of, among many others, John Locke, John Stuart Mill and Adam Smith, is freedom. Most important are individual sovereignty and negative freedoms. Within the constraints of the law, what individuals choose to do with their liberty is up to them. Political liberalism has been the foundation of politics and policy in the USA since the nation was first established.

A strong version of neo-liberalism in the economic sphere was especially apparent in the USA's uncompromising free-market policies during the latter part of the twentieth century. Its political manifestation can be seen in the emergence of political movements such as the right-wing libertarian Tea Party group within the Republican party, who call for, among other things, lower taxes and reductions in public spending. This is based on the liberal principle that no one should be coerced into surrendering their private property for the good of society.

5.2 Constitutional Settings of Well-being

This section reviews the constitutions and other important political texts of the USA and Canada, with the objective of identifying the central principles and values that characterise the political settings of well-being in the two countries.

5.2.1 USA (1789, Rev. 1992)

The American Declaration of Independence (1776) famously enshrined the "inalienable rights" of "Life, Liberty and the pursuit of happiness." This historic document provided the basis of the constitution of the USA (1789, rev. 1992), whose preamble states that the constitution is established in order to "promote the general Welfare, and secure the Blessings of Liberty to ourselves and our Posterity." It is also the foundation of the American Declaration of the Rights and Duties of Man (1948), whose preamble states that "All men are born free and equal, in dignity and in rights." The liberal theme continues in the Charter of the Organization of American States, of which the USA is the largest and most influential member: the Charter opens with the statement that "the historic mission of America is to offer to man a land of liberty and a favorable environment for the development of his personality and the realization of his just aspirations... within the framework of democratic institutions, of a system of individual liberty and social justice based on respect for the essential rights of man."

The constitution reiterates the importance of individual freedom and rights in numerous places, including in Amendment V to the preamble to the Bill of Rights: No person shall "be deprived of life, liberty, or property, without due process of law; nor shall private property be taken for public use, without just compensation." The rights included in the constitution overlap to some extent with the International Bill of Rights: civil and political rights are strongly protected; for example, the rights to life and to own property (A.XIV.1); to a fair trial (A.VI); and to freedom of speech, religion and assembly (A.I). Others are added (a controversial example being Amendment II on the right to bear arms). Many of the social, economic and cultural rights of the IBHR, however, are omitted from the national constitution (although may be included in some individual state constitutions): for example, health and healthcare, education, and social protection and an adequate standard of living are not included as rights.

Together, these instruments express a version of classical liberalism: Liberty is the foundational value, and should be promoted through the protection of the rights of citizens against the state. This type of liberalism involves predominantly negative rights of non-interference, based on the inalienable sovereignty of the individual. Liberalism in this sense was designed to liberate individuals from repressive traditions, customs and social hierarchies. It is from here that the fundamental value of the individual as his own sovereign entity emerges.

5.2.2 *Canada (1867, Rev. 1992)*

The Constitution of Canada is also strongly influenced by political liberalism. Part 1 of the Canadian Constitution Act (1982) is entitled "Canadian Charter of Rights and Freedoms," and begins with four "Fundamental Freedoms": Freedom of conscience and religion (1.B2,a); Freedom of thought, belief, opinion and expression, including freedom of the press and other media of communication (1.B2,b); Freedom of peaceful assembly (1.B2,c); and Freedom of association (1.B2,d). The Charter also enshrines a set of democratic rights (1.C), Mobility rights (1.D), Legal rights (1.E), and a statement of Equality in these rights (1.F).

Like that of its larger neighbour, this political conception of the good affirms Liberty as the basic value, to be protected by treating individuals as rights-bearers. Indeed, the Liberal Party of Canada dominated Canadian politics in the twentieth century. However, compared to the USA, Canadian liberalism arguably has a more detailed conception of the necessary conditions of freedom, demonstrated by social policies such as universal healthcare.

Despite many contemporary differences in culture and public policy regimes, the USA and Canada share a historic and modern agenda of political liberalism.

5.2.3 *The Second Wave of Well-being in North America*

Beyond these codified political and legal instruments, the Beyond GDP "second wave" has brought well-being into political discourses in new ways in North America, most prominently in Canada. The Canadian Index of Wellbeing (CIW), developed and hosted by a team at the University of Waterloo, is comprised by eight domains, listed below with illustrative examples of sub-domains and measurement indicators:

- Community Vitality
  - Social relationships, Social norms and values
- Democratic Engagement
  - Participation in politics, Political environment
- Education
  - Educational attainment, Knowledge and skills

- Environment
  - Natural resources
- Healthy Populations
  - Physical and mental health, Healthcare provision
- Leisure and Culture
  - Participation in the arts, Participation in social and physical recreational activities, Vacations
- Living Standards
  - Income and wealth, Income Inequality, Economic security, Food security
- Time Use
  - Work, Commuting, Socialising, Sleep, Time pressure

Based on an "ongoing cycle of public engagement, consultation and refinement" about what Canadians believe to be most important in life, the CIW aims to be a dynamic approach to tracking national well-being, while remaining faithful to the original "Canadian values" on which it is based (CIW 2016, p. 16). The index covers the same ground as the OECD Better Life index, except for the omission in the CIW of *Life Satisfaction*, although the *Healthy Populations* domain includes an indicator of self-reported mental health.

In the USA, the United States Census Bureau provides official statistics from social surveys including the American Community Survey, the American Housing Survey, and the Survey of Income and Program Participation.[1] A number of domains of these surveys relate to individual, household and community well-being. A selection of domains is listed below, along with sub-domains and examples of measurement indicators from across the different surveys:

[1] https://www.census.gov/programs-surveys/acs, https://www.census.gov/topics.html, accessed 10 February 2019.

- Income and Poverty
  - Household income and wealth, Income inequality, Public Assistance, Food security (use of food stamps)
- Housing
  - Home ownership, Physical and financial characteristics of homes, Living space, Privacy, Self-reported "favorable housing conditions."
- Education
  - Educational Attainment, School enrolment, Satisfaction with schools
- Employment
  - Employment status, Occupation, Weeks and hours worked, Commuting time
- Families and living arrangements
  - Marital status, Family composition, Child care and elder care
- Health
  - Health insurance coverage, Disability, Fertility, Prevalence of HIV/AIDS
- Neighbourhood conditions and community services
  - Neighbourhood safety
  - Percent of households reporting favourable neighbourhood conditions
- Public Sector
  - Voting, Satisfaction with community services

These surveys and domains are not brought together explicitly as a framework of "well-being," and measurement does not guarantee policy action. However, the fact of their measurement does represent a recognition within the US federal government that "The living standards of households are traditionally measured by income. However, income is not the only measure available. Extended measures of well-being help deepen our knowledge about household conditions in ways not captured by money alone" (Rogers and Ryan 2007, p. 1).

5.3 Mass Priorities in North America

The discussion so far has focused on conceptions of the good in the political arena. Table 5.1 shows findings from the World Values Survey about the mass priorities of the civilian populations of North America.

Table 5.1 shows that, within the politically liberal institutional environment in which they live, people in North America tend to prioritise their social relationships, with family and friends most likely to be rated as "Very important" in both the USA and Canada. A similar proportion in both countries believes leisure time to be very important, and the domain of Politics is universally deprioritised. The main difference between the two countries, then, is in the relative prioritisation of religion and work, with religion more important to citizens of the USA, and work more important to Canadians.

While these country-level findings smooth over many individual, regional and national differences, they do reveal mass priorities at the population level. In both countries, political and legal institutions are structured around the primary importance of individual liberty. At the level of citizens, the World Values Survey suggests that this liberty is used principally in pursuit of social relationships. Overall, this implies that the principles of political liberalism do not necessarily translate into a devaluation of sociality.

Table 5.1 Value priorities in the USA and Canada (% "Very important")

USA		*Canada*	
Family	94.6	Family	92.8
Friends	59.7	Friends	63.1
Religion	47.4	Work	48.6
Leisure time	37.7	Leisure time	40.8
Work	32.6	Religion	32.0
Politics	11.0	Politics	11.7

Note The most recent data at the time of writing (Wave 6) are not available for Canada, so Wave 5 (2005–2009) is used for both countries
Source World Values Survey, Wave 5 (Ingelehart et al. 2014)

5.4 Chapter Summary

Political liberalism provides the basis of political conceptions of the good in North America, with individual freedom as the defining principle. This liberalism is manifested differently in the USA and Canada, with more policy focus on social and economic rights in Canada. Despite worries about the individualism inherent in classical liberalism, findings suggest that, in practice, liberalism does not necessarily entail the devaluation of sociality; social relationships are a mass priority in both countries. Common priorities emerging from second wave initiatives (broadly conceived) include Material living standards, Work, Education, Health and Communities and families. As we are beginning to see, these are common constituents of conceptions of the good in many other cultures.

References

CIW. (2016). *How are Canadians Really Doing? The 2016 CIW National Report.* Waterloo, ON: Canadian Index of Wellbeing and University of Waterloo.

Inglehart, R., Haerpfer,C., Moreno, A., Welzel, C., Kizilova, K., Diez-Medrano, J., et al. (Eds.). (2014). *World Values Survey: Round Six—Country-Pooled Datafile Version.* www.worldvaluessurvey.org/WVSDocumentationWV6.jsp. Madrid: JD Systems Institute.

Rogers, A. L., & Ryan, C. L. (2007). *Extended Measures of Well-Being: Living Conditions in the United States, 2003.* Washington, DC: US Census Bureau. https://www.census.gov/prod/2007pubs/p70-110.pdf. Accessed 10 February 2019.

CHAPTER 6

Well-being in Latin America

Abstract This chapter presents evidence from Latin America in relation to the core principles and values of the political settings of well-being in the region. First, the Latin American *Buen Vivir* approach to well-being is discussed, and links to other approaches to well-being (such as Aristotelian ethics and Communitarianism) are explored. Next, the constitutions of a selection of Latin American countries are examined, with the aim of identifying the central principles of political conceptions of well-being. Evidence from the World Values Survey provides another perspective on the mass priorities of different countries in this region. The Latin American philosophy of *buen vivir* is a conception of the good that sees human beings as one part of a complex system of life, and human well-being as co-extensive with the well-being of the entire system. The *buen vivir* philosophy is based on radically different assumptions to conceptions of the good found elsewhere. Social relationships, the Natural environment, and connection to a higher dimension of truth and spirituality are the cornerstone values of *buen vivir*. The World Values Survey shows that social relationships, particularly family relationships, are at the heart of well-being in the countries studied.

Keywords Latin America · Values · Well-being · *Buen Vivir*

A. Austin, *A Universal Declaration of Human Well-being*,
Wellbeing in Politics and Policy,
https://doi.org/10.1007/978-3-030-27107-7_6

This chapter presents evidence from Latin America. First, the Latin American *Buen Vivir* approach to well-being is discussed. Then, the constitutions of a selection of Latin American countries are examined, with the aim of identifying the core principles and values of the political settings of well-being in these places. Evidence from the World Values Survey provides another perspective on the mass priorities of different countries in this region.

6.1 *Buen Vivir*: A Philosophy of Well-being

Buen vivir is a philosophy of life. It is used as an umbrella term for a set of social movements that have gained mainstream policy traction in some Latin American countries, particularly the Andean countries of Bolivia and Ecuador, whose national constitutions have explicitly incorporated the principles of *buen vivir*. The Spanish term translates as "Good living," and encapsulates an idea that is expressed in different indigenous languages across the continent, from Chile to Venezuela (Gudynas 2011; Rodríguez 2016). Although there is variation in social movements in different communities and countries, the *Buen Vivir* philosophy is the common foundation of them all.

Buen vivir is an alternative ontology of human being, involving a conception of the good that is profoundly different to most Western ideals. The Bolivian Constitution describes it as a "holistic concept based on complementarity, solidarity, harmony and collective well-being."[1] The subject of the harmonious collective life is the extended community of all human beings, other living beings and nature. On this view, the natural environment is not something separate to human life; humans are just one constitutive part of a great social-ecological-cosmological system. Nature is not instrumental to human well-being; instead, well-being and harms are shared.

Another noteworthy aspect of *Buen Vivir* is its inherent conception of time. An important value is the relationship of humans to ancestors, and ancestral knowledge, values and culture. The present is deeply connected to the past and also to future generations, but history is not a linear process, it is a cycle of the totality of life, in its widest sense. On this view, well-being

[1] Constitution of Bolivia (2009). Retrieved from https://constituteproject.org/constitution/Bolivia_2009.pdf?lang=en (accessed January 2019).

is a (non-linear) way of being, not an outcome. A good life consists of co-existing in ongoing relationships of deep communion with fellow humans, other living beings, and the natural environment.

The Bolivian articulation of *Buen Vivir* derives from the *Aymara* concept of *suma qamaña*, which means "to live in plenitude" (Rodríguez 2016, p. 279). Plenitude here does not refer to quantities of material goods, but to the quality of relationships within the Great Community—the dense network of relationships across time and space between all elements of the natural world and the cosmos: the "spatial-temporal-harmonious totality of existence" Walsh (2010, p. 18).

The idea of a good life as a flourishing, fruitful, abundant life is found in Aristotelian ethics. For Aristotle, the master value of human life is *Eudaimonia*—living a good, successful life in the social world. Again, this cannot be measured by quantities of material goods, but refers to flourishing as a human; enjoying the bounty of a full human life by excelling in those capabilities that make humans truly human. It is interesting to note that the word *eudaimon* can equally be used to describe a particularly productive or fruitful tree, or indeed any kind of abundance.[2]

The *Buen Vivir* philosophy has clear links to the Aristotelian, communitarian conception of the person as a social animal embedded in a multidimensional social setting (Sect. 2.3). *Buen vivir*, however, is not only concerned with social setting, but extends the contextual setting of well-being to include the natural environment. A further extension of the contextual setting of *Buen vivir* is the inclusion of a spiritual dimension. This recalls the idea of a "community of memory" (Bellah et al. 1993), disparate groups of people who share values, histories, identities and memories. The dimension of *Buen Vivir* that emphasises connections to the ancestral past and the wisdom of ancestors is a paradigmatic example of a community of memory, in this case perhaps better described as a "community of spirituality," or more generally as a "community of values." A community of values is an important aspect of the ethical reasoning and practice of its members: it is part of both the practical reasoning and practical action aspects of Integrity (Sect. 3.2). As we saw in Part I, the idea of connection with a source of meaning and value beyond one's immediate sensory experience is a good that has emerged across tradition, geography and time.

[2]Personal communication.

Although translation into modern English or Spanish loses many of the nuances of *buen vivir* as it is traditionally articulated, and although *buen vivir* is not a single uniform view, we can say that the fundamental values of *buen vivir* in general include: Social relationships (to close family and community, to the institutions of society, and to the human family at the most general level); relationships with nature; and relationships to a dimension of spirituality or divinity in terms of transcendent wisdom and knowledge about the grand totality of existence. *Buen vivir* is therefore a thoroughly relational conception of the good, on which well-being is determined by the quality of the inter-relationships that constitute the whole complex system.

6.2 Constitutional Settings of Well-being: *Buen Vivir* in Politics and Policy

In this section the constitutions of Bolivia and Ecuador are reviewed, with the objective of identifying the main principles and values of the political settings of well-being in these countries.

6.2.1 Bolivia

Bolivia has been at the forefront of incorporating the principles of *Buen vivir* into national politics and policy. The preamble of the national constitution states that "We have left the colonial, republican and neo-liberal State in the past. We take on the historic challenge of collectively constructing a Unified Social State of Pluri-National Communitarian law…" Article 8 goes on to affirm that the State is based on "the values of unity, equality, inclusion, dignity, liberty, solidarity, reciprocity, respect, interdependence, harmony, transparency, equilibrium, equality of opportunity, social and gender equality in participation, common welfare, responsibility, social justice, distribution and redistribution of the social wealth and assets for well-being." The emphasis on "solidarity," "Communitarian law," "social justice" and "social wealth" sets a distinctly social tone, reflecting the fundamental principles of *Buen vivir*.

The constitution sets out a guarantee of "access of all people to education, health and work" (Art.9.5). "Fundamental rights" include the right to water and food (Art.16.I), which includes a constitutional guarantee of food security, "by means of healthy, adequate and sufficient food for the entire population" (Art.16.II). Also included under the heading of

Fundamental Rights is the right to a decent home (Art.19), which "dignifies family and community life." Particularly stressed are "Environmental Rights" of "a healthy, protected and balanced environment," which must be "granted to individuals and collectives of present and future generations, as well as to other living things" (Art.33). The focus on sociality and the natural environment is continued in a more detailed articulation of the right to Education, whose stated objectives are "the full development of persons and the strengthening of social conscience that is critical in and for life. Education shall be directed towards the following: individual and collective development; the development of the competencies, attitudes, and physical and intellectual skills that link theory to productive practice; the conservation and protection of the environment, biodiversity and the land to assure well-being" (Art.80).

The examples above show that, while human rights apply to every individual, the themes of *Buen Vivir* of collective well-being, harmony, equilibrium and solidarity run through them all. The theme of environmental protection is ever-present. The explicit rejection in the preamble of (neo)-liberalism, in favour of communitarian values, is the basis of a detailed articulation of substantive positive rights and positive duties of the state.

6.2.2 Ecuador

Ecuador is another country that has embraced the principles of B*uen vivir* at the highest levels of politics. The preamble to the constitution refers explicitly to *Buen Vivir*, declaring the ambition to build "A new form of public coexistence, in diversity and in harmony with nature, to achieve the good way of living, the *sumak kawsay* [...based on] the celebration of nature, the Pacha Mama (Mother Earth), of which we are a part and is vital to our existence."

In another explicit reference to traditional philosophy, Chapter VII of the constitution is entitled "The System of *Buen Vivir.*" It describes a "coordinated set of systems, institutions, policies, norms, programs and services" designed to underpin and enable the rights enshrined in the Constitution (Art.340), which include the standard social, economic, cultural, civil and political rights found in international law, plus a set of environmental rights. As in the Bolivian constitution, this demonstrates an ambition to uphold the rights of individuals and communities through the development of a social setting based on ecological-communitarian values. Liberty is to be achieved through solidarity. The aspiration is to foster these values through formal institutional measures—policies, programmes and services—as well as through the informal institutions of social norms. The political setting of well-being is conceived here as an interconnected system of institutions.

Although the principles of *buen vivir* are written into the constitutions of Bolivia and Ecuador, criticism has been aimed at the governments of these countries for failing to implement them in reality. A common source of this perceived failure is the pull of the income that can be earned through the extractive industries. Critics claim that constitutional commitments to environmental protection have been sacrificed for the sake of a capitalist drive for national income, thereby disregarding the *Buen vivir* philosophy, which aims to be an alternative to modern capitalism (e.g. Van Teijlingen and Hogenboom 2016). A further criticism is that the modern *buen vivir* movement wrongly sees *buen vivir* as a homogenous concept, whereas in reality, it is articulated quite differently across different indigenous communities (e.g. Villalba 2013). It seems that some feel that *buen vivir* has been co-opted by political elites, homogenised and detached from its roots in the alternative worldviews of indigenous cultures.

6.3 Mass Priorities in Latin America

The discussion so far has focused on philosophical and political conceptions of the good. We now turn to the mass priorities of civilian populations. Table 6.1 shows data from the World Values Survey (Inglehart et al. 2014) for a selection of Latin American countries.

Table 6.1 shows the familiar pattern of Family being most likely to be rated as "Very important," and Politics least likely. As in other regions, social relationships are prioritised, although here, this domain is clearly divided into family and friends, with family relationships taking top priority in each country. A possible explanation for this is that, as in other countries (e.g. the post-communist countries of Eastern Europe) where, in recent history, authoritarian regimes dismantled and undermined the institutions of civil society, the bonds of family are particularly important (e.g. Burt 2016).

It is also notable that, in these countries, Work is rated as particularly important. A tentative explanation of this is that work is a proxy for material resources in these countries. As well as these commonalities, though, there are important differences across the countries; for example, the domain of Religion is "very important" for less than a third of Argentinians, but around two-thirds of Ecuadorians. However, the utmost importance of family across the region is undeniable.

Table 6.1 Value priorities in a selection of Latin American countries (% "Very important")

Argentina		*Brazil*		*Chile*		*Colombia*		*Ecuador*	
Family	88.9	Family	87.4	Family	91.7	Family	85.1	Family	98.6
Work	57.4	Work	63.6	Work	56.3	Work	76.3	Work	88.5
Friends	53.9	Religion	51.5	Leisure time	56.1	Religion	58.9	Religion	67.1
Religion	24.1	Friends	33.0	Friends	35.1	Leisure time	49.4	Leisure time	55.9
Leisure time	33.7	Leisure time	32.8	Religion	23.8	Friends	30.7	Friends	32.6
Politics	8.3	Politics	12.5	Politics	7.4	Politics	9.8	Politics	21.1

Source World Values Survey, Wave 6 (Inglehart et al. 2014)

6.4 Chapter Summary

The *buen vivir* philosophy is a conception of the good that sees human beings as one part of an all-encompassing complex system of life, and human well-being as co-extensive with the well-being of the entire system. Despite criticisms and concerns about implementation at the political and policy levels by those governments who have, on paper, adopted it, it remains the case that the *buen vivir* philosophy is based on radically different assumptions to conceptions of the good found elsewhere. At the same time, however, connections can be made to familiar strands of political theory, particularly communitarianism and environmental ethics. There are also connections to the co-living movements of northern Europe (Chapter 4). Social relationships, the Natural environment, and connection to a higher dimension of truth and spirituality are the cornerstone values of *buen vivir*.

References

Bellah, R. N., Madsen, R., Sullivan, W. M., Swidler, A., & Tipton, S. M. (1993). Habits of the heart: Individualism and commitment in American life. *Journal of Leisure Research, 25*(1), 100.

Burt, J. (2016). *Political Violence and the Authoritarian State in Peru: Silencing Civil Society*. Basingstoke: Palgrave Macmillan.

Gudynas, E. (2011). Buen Vivir: Today's tomorrow. *Development, 54*(4), 441–447.

Inglehart, R., Haerpfer, C., Moreno, A., Welzel, C., Kizilova, K., Diez-Medrano, J., et al. (Eds.). (2014). *World Values Survey: Round Six—Country-Pooled Datafile Version*. http://www.worldvaluessurvey.org/WVSDocumentationWV6.jsp. Madrid: JD Systems Institute.

Rodríguez, I. (2016). Historical reconstruction and cultural identity building as a local pathway to 'living well' amongst the Pemon of Venezuela. In S. White & C. Blackmore (Eds.), *Cultures of Wellbeing* (pp. 260–280). London: Palgrave Macmillan.

Van Teijlingen, K., & Hogenboom, B. (2016). Debating alternative development at the mining frontier: Buen Vivir and the conflict around el Mirador Mine in Ecuador. *Journal of Developing Societies, 32*(4), 382–420.

Villalba, U. (2013). Buen Vivir vs development: A paradigm shift in the Andes? *Third World Quarterly, 34*(8), 1427–1442.

Walsh, C. (2010). Development as Buen Vivir: Institutional arrangements and (de)colonial entanglements. *Development, 53*(1), 15–21.

CHAPTER 7

Well-being in Asia

Abstract This chapter presents evidence about the central principles and values of political conceptions of well-being in countries in East, South, West and Central Asia. First, traditional Confucian, Daoist, Hindu and Arabic conceptions of the good are discussed, and areas of overlap with other ethical theories are explored. Next, the national constitutions of a selection of countries are examined, and findings from the World Values Survey give a broad view of mass priorities in different regions. In the midst of great surface-level diversity, common threads emerge from the various philosophical traditions and modern socio-political settings. Communitarian values are widespread: the centrality of social and community relationships in the good life is expressed in multiple ways. Protection of cultural heritage and participation in cultural life are ubiquitous features of the constitutions. This may be interpreted as the good of belonging to a social group with whom one shares identities, interests and ends. A final theme to emerge is the good of contemplation and connection to a "higher" dimension of meaning and value, sometimes achieved through religious and spiritual practices. In sum, Social relationships, Cultural participation, and the Contemplative life are common features of the ethical traditions discussed in this chapter.

Keywords Values · Well-being · Asia · Communitarian values

A. Austin, *A Universal Declaration of Human Well-being*,
Wellbeing in Politics and Policy,
https://doi.org/10.1007/978-3-030-27107-7_7

This chapter presents evidence from countries in East, South, West and Central Asia. First, Confucian, Daoist, Hindu and Arabic conceptions of the good are discussed, and areas of overlap with other ethical theories are explored. Next, the national constitutions of a selection of countries are examined, with the aim of identifying the central principles of modern political conceptions of the good. Findings from the World Values Survey give a broad view of mass priorities in different regions of the continent.

7.1 Confucian, Daoist, Hindu and Arabic Conceptions of the Good

Chapter 3 demonstrated parallels between Confucian, Hindu, and Ancient Greek ethics. To recap, each of these traditions includes a variant of what we know as virtue ethics: To live a good life is to be a good person; being a good person consists in the possession and practice of particular virtues. Furthermore, there were significant commonalities in the substantive virtues advocated. The following sections examine the conceptions of the good inherent in these and other ethical theories found across Asia.

7.1.1 *Chinese Ethics: Confucian and Daoist Conceptions of the Good*

Although Confucius never set out a single definitive set of virtues, his collected works—the Analects (Ames and Rosemont 1998)—can be mined to elicit those character traits and dispositions that he saw as indispensable to living a good life. The core Confucian values are commonly summarised as *jen* (humanity, benevolence); *yi* (good, mutually respectful social relationships, starting with the family and extending outwards); *li* (propriety, temperance, courteous observance of etiquette and rites); *zhi* (nurturing and exercising virtue); and *xin* (truthfulness and sincerity in the practical application of the other virtues) (Cleary 1992; Huang 1997; Yao and Yao 2000). Others have detected an additional Confucian virtue, labelled as "Transcendence" and defined as "Strengths that forge connections to the larger universe and thereby provide meaning [to life]" (Dahlsgaard et al. 2005, p. 205).

The Confucian virtues are manifested in a person who cares for others, and who enjoys good and mutually respectful social relationships, partly due to his close understanding and observance of the rules and norms of his social setting. He is temperate, in that he takes the middle way between extremes of character. He is practically wise: he employs the right virtues in the right situations. His well-being is also constituted by his capacity for contemplation and connection to a transcendent dimension.

This (very simplified) account of Confucian virtue ethics demonstrates many similarities with Aristotelian ethics. It has been suggested that the Chinese *Dao* (the way to becoming a good person) and the Greek *Eudaimonia* (flourishing) play a similar role in their respective ethical traditions (Yu 2007). In addition to the shared substantive virtues of Benevolence and Justice, Confucius and Aristotle both defined virtue as a moderate path (the "mean") between extremes in particular spheres of virtue (NE 1106a26–b28; Haberman 1998a), and advised that virtue be developed by observing the conduct of "exemplary persons." Both Aristotle and Confucius saw ethics as the practical science of being and doing well in the social world: Aristotle's organising principle of *phronesis* (practical wisdom) is similar to the Confucian ideal of *xin*—excellence in the practical application of virtue. For both, virtue is (in fact, can only be) developed and realised in a social context: well-being (the good life) is deeply relational.

An alternative Chinese ethic is found in Daoism, as articulated in the *Daodejing* and the *Zhuangzi* associated with the philosophers Laozi and Zhuangzi (c.sixth–third century BCE) (Wong 2018). A central feature of Daoist ethics is the conception of human life as one small part of a much larger sphere of existence. Human well-being requires harmonious relationships with the rest of humanity, and the natural world, in the context of the entire cosmos (Wong 2018). Understanding, attunement, and gentle responsiveness to this great interconnected system are at the heart of a good life. The *Daodejing* advocates a way of life involving receptivity and compassion, simplicity and sincerity, and softness and gentleness (Nelson 2009, p. 303). Kindness and thoughtfulness are central to this tradition.

Given its expansive concept of life and being that includes the natural, non-human world, Daoism has also been interpreted as providing a basis for environmental ethics (e.g. Chan 2009; Nelson 2009). These features are shared with the Latin American *Buen Vivir* philosophy discussed in Chapter 6. Like *Buen Vivir*, Daoist ethics is relational not only in terms of the social relationality characteristic of Aristotelian and Confucian ethics, but also in terms of relationships with the great entirety of existence. The Daoist idea of unforced, harmonious connection with the human and non-human world is contrary to oppression and subordination of others (other humans, non-human animals and the natural world). From the point of view of maintaining good relationships between humans, this implies that a well (justly) governed state (insofar as a state is required) is another crucial aspect of well-being.

7.1.2 *Indian Ethics: Hindu Conceptions of the Good*

While "Hindu philosophy" is an umbrella term for a range of Indian schools of thought across geography and time, some central themes can be identified. As we saw in Chapter 3, like Aristotle and Confucius, the ancient Hindu tradition employed a version of virtue ethics, with virtue to be developed in the social world, through practical experience and learning from exemplary virtuous people (e.g. *Apastambadharmasutra* 1.20.6–8, cited in Hacker 2006). On this view, living a good life is living in accordance with virtue. Core Hindu virtues that emerge from the sacred texts, the *Vedas* and the *Upanishads* (some of which date back to the same era in which Aristotle, Confucius and Laozi were developing their ethical theories), include courage, justice, benevolence, temperance, wisdom and transcendence (Dahlsgaard et al. 2005). This set of characteristics of the good person is strongly reminiscent of the Greek and Chinese virtues. This shows that both the procedure for identifying virtues (learn from good people), and the substantive virtues thereby identified, are common across these different traditions.

A central concept of Hindu ethics is *brahman*—roughly, the interconnectedness of everything with everything (Haberman 1998b). As in the Latin American and Daoist traditions, in addition to the practical application of virtue in the social world, an important aspect of the good life is striving to attain a higher or transcendental knowledge of the self as a part of, and in relation to, this great interconnected system of everything. As in the other traditions, the great system of everything incorporates time: a clear expression of this in the Hindu tradition is the concept of the ongoing cycle of birth and rebirth (*karma*). The attainment of this higher knowledge of the self as part of the great spatio-temporal system of existence is the pinnacle of well-being. The good life is lived by the person who strives towards this aim: as for Aristotle, well-being is a process, not a state.

7.1.3 *Arabic Conceptions of the Good*

Insights from the ancient Arabic schools of thought can be found in texts attributed to the thinkers Al-Fārābī, Avicenna and Averroes. Based on a set of metaphysical premises particular to this tradition, these ancient Arabic scholars viewed the good life ("happiness") as being obtained through the conjunction of the human intellect (or mind) with a higher wisdom or knowledge—the "active intellect." Attainment of this blending of the self with the higher source of meaning and value requires a contemplative life (Hasse 2018). On this view, knowledge of and connection to a transcendental source of knowledge, meaning and value is the ultimate value of human life.

The religious life is of central importance in the Arabic tradition. The "five pillars of Islam" are *Shahada* (Testimony of Faith), *Salat* (regular prayer), *Zakat* (charity, giving alms), *Ramadan* (fasting) and *Hajj* (pilgrimage). The active practice of the Islamic faith in everyday life includes compassion and benevolence (*Zakat*) as a central tenet. As in the other traditions discussed here, traditional Arabic conceptions of the good affirm a way of life that includes kindness to others and contemplation of a "higher" good or truth.

The accounts set out above demonstrate areas of overlap between ancient Chinese, Indian, Arabic Greek and Latin American conceptions of the good. It is striking that accounts of what it means to live well that were developed in such distant regions, traditions and times came to some similar conclusions about the basics of a good human life. Common themes include the importance of two kinds of relationality. First, across these traditions we find that mutually respectful family and community relationships are an integral part of well-being. There was also some convergence in the virtues and practices that enable a person to live well in the social world: Benevolence and Justice are common proposals. Second, connection with a realm of truth and value beyond the human world is at the centre of well-being. This is expressed variously as connections with ancestors and ancestral wisdom, contemplation of truth, mindfulness and connections to the divine. To summarise, lessons in well-being from the Asian traditions include the importance of harmonious social relationships and a contemplative approach to life.

7.2 Constitutional Settings of Well-being

Moving on from traditional approaches, this section examines the modern constitutions of a selection of countries across East Asia (Bhutan and

China), West Asia (Qatar) and South Asia (India). The objective is to identify the main political principles and values that provide the parameters of the settings of well-being in these different places.

7.2.1 Bhutan (2008)

As a forerunner of the second wave of well-being, the constitution of Bhutan is a testament to the Beyond GDP movement.

The preamble to the constitution pledges to "enhance the unity, happiness and well-being of the people for all time." A central Principle of State Policy is to "promote those conditions that will enable the pursuit of Gross National Happiness" (Art.9.2). The constitution sets out a number of domains relevant to this. After statements relating to the form of government (a democratic constitutional monarchy), Articles 3–5 concern Spiritual Heritage, Culture, and Environment. Beginning with the spiritual life, the constitution states that "Buddhism is the spiritual heritage of Bhutan, which promotes the principles and values of peace, non-violence, compassion and tolerance" (Art.3.1). With regard to cultural life, the state will "preserve, protect and promote the cultural heritage of the country," including monuments and sacred sites, the arts, language and "local arts, custom, knowledge, and culture" (4.3). To reinforce the latter, the state will ensure "the continued evolution of traditional values and institutions" (4.2). In relation to the environment, "Every Bhutanese is a trustee of the Kingdom's natural resources and environment for the benefit of the present and future generations." This emphasis on Environment shows that well-being is anchored in the natural world.

As in other places, the good life is conceived as one that draws upon history, heritage and tradition. The opening articles of the constitution make it clear that the spiritual life is a defining feature of the Bhutanese political-social-cultural context—that is, a central aspect of the "conditions that will enable the pursuit of Gross National Happiness." State protection and support are guaranteed for traditional values and customs. However, "culture" is not defined as static, but as "an evolving dynamic force" (4.2), whereby traditions evolve in a way that is "sustainable as a progressive society" (4.2). Traditional values and institutions are advocated as a sound foundation of modern Bhutanese political and social culture, and of the Bhutanese political vision of well-being and progress.

To promote this vision of an alternative model, the Bhutanese Gross National Happiness Index was developed, composed of the nine domains of

Psychological Well-being, Health, Education, Time Use, Cultural Diversity and Resilience, Good Governance, Community Vitality, Ecological Diversity and Resilience, and Living Standards (Ura et al. 2012). There is a clear overlap between the index and the principles set out in the constitution. As a pioneer of the Beyond GDP movement, the influence of Bhutan's approach on "second wave" initiatives across the world is clear (compare, for example, the Canadian Index of Well-being).

7.2.2 *China (1982, Rev. 2004)*

In keeping with the Confucian principle of reverence for the past and ancestors, the Preamble to the Constitution of The People's Republic of China begins with the observation that China has "one of the longest histories in the world" and "a splendid culture." It continues by setting out a modern history of the nation, including important political figures, and describes its vision of a socialist state guided by the principles of Equality, Unity and Mutual assistance. A central aim of the state is to increase economic productivity and to "improve the material and cultural life of the people" (Art.14). State policy concerns include the domains of Education (from pre-school to adult education) (Art.19–20), Health and healthcare, through the promotion of both modern and traditional Chinese medicine (Art.21), and access to and participation in Culture (Art.22). The Confucian value of *li* (observance of etiquette, tradition and social rules) is expressed in the stated aim of "...promoting the formulation and observance of rules of conduct..." (Art.24). Also included in the State's purview is Protection of the natural environment (Art.26).

The Chinese constitution can be interpreted as the statement of an ambition to blend modernity and tradition. This can be seen in the sections relating to the Economy, Education, Health and Culture. The rights found in the International Bill of Human Rights are included in the constitution (Chapter II), with many translated into language consistent with the political and economic socialism set out in the first part of the document (Art.1–18). For example, the right to work is expressed as follows: "Work is the glorious duty of every able-bodied citizen. All working people in State-owned enterprises and in urban and rural economic collectives should perform their tasks with an attitude consonant with their status as masters of the country..." (Art.42). In sum, the Chinese political conception of the good is based on strongly communitarian principles, with citizens who are educated and healthy such that they can contribute to collective welfare.

7.2.3 *India (1949, Rev. 2016)*

The preamble of the Indian constitution sets out the fundamental principles of Justice, Liberty, Equality and Fraternity that should underpin the social, economic and political environment. Part IV enumerates the "Directive Principles of the State." The first of these is the ambition to "secure a social order for the promotion of the welfare of the people" (Art.38).

Central policy principles for the achievement of this setting include provisions relating to Material resources, livelihoods and wealth (Art.39.a–d), Health (Art.39.e–f, 47), access to Political power through strong local government (Art.40), Work (Art.41–43), Education (Art.41, 45, 46) and Social security (Art.41). Protection of the natural environment is a duty of the state (Art.48A), as is protection of "monuments, and places and objects of national importance" (Art.49). In addition to the basic rights of the IBHR, "Fundamental Duties" of all citizens include the responsibility to "promote harmony and the spirit of brotherhood among all the people of India" (51A.e), and "to strive towards excellence in all spheres of individual and collective activity…" (51A.j). The emphasis on unity, solidarity, non-violence and harmony can be traced back to the modern history of the nation, but also resonates with ancient Hindu ethics.

Overall, the Indian constitution sets out a vision of a society based on justice in the social, economic and political spheres, as the setting of well-being. The domains of Social relationships, Material resources, Education, Health, Work, Natural environment and Cultural heritage receive particular attention. As in Bhutan and China, well-being includes being able to benefit from a rich national history and heritage, and participate in ongoing cultural life. Sharing in a collective identity is part of the good life.

7.2.4 *Qatar (2003) and the United Arab Emirates*

Modern Arabic political conceptions of the good society and the good life often combine traditional religious ethics with modern political concepts; for example, like many Arab nations, Qatar is a signatory to the Cairo Declaration on Human Rights in Islam (1990), a statement of the ways in which fundamental rights and duties are expressed within the Islamic religion.

The constitution of Qatar opens with the statement that "Qatar is an Arab State, sovereign and independent. Its religion is Islam, and the Islamic

Law is the main source of its legislations" (Art.1). Chapter II sets out "The basic pillars of Society," which are "Justice, Charity, Freedom, Equality, and Good morals" (Art.18). As well as maintaining security and stability (Art.19), the state "strives to consolidate the spirit of national unity, solidarity, and fraternity among all citizens" (Art.20), with family as "the nucleus of society" (Art.21).

Within the framework of the basic pillars, particular domains singled out for state support include Public Health (Art.23); Cultural Life, including "science, literature, arts and national cultural heritage" (Art.24); Education (Art.25); Living standards and Work (Art.28), and the Natural Environment (Art.33). Special mention is made of young people, who are constitutionally protected against "exploitation...[and] physical, mental and spiritual neglect" (Art.22). Chapter III sets out Public Rights and Duties, based on the Cairo Declaration of Human Rights in Islam.

The main body of the constitution includes a legal framework for economic governance, which stipulates that the natural wealth of Qatar (large oil and natural gas reserves) be managed "...on the basis of social justice...to achieve economic and social development, production increase, realizing prosperity for the citizens, raising their living standard, providing work opportunities for them..." (Art.28). Material living standards and Work are important constituents of the Qatari conception of well-being.

The setting of well-being in Qatar is characterised by a high-income economy, a monarchic political environment, and a small population which includes a majority of expatriates and a multitude of cultural influences, from ancient Bedouin culture to modern global capitalism. Overall, the constitution sets out an institutional framework designed to promote a conception of the good in which the religious life and the family are the most important aspects of well-being, along with the additional priorities of Health, Education, Work and Cultural Life.

7.2.5 *United Arab Emirates*

In the United Arab Emirates (UAE), as in Qatar, the Islamic religion provides the foundation of law and society, and the guiding principles of the good life (constitution Preamble, articles 7, 12). The clearest articulation of an Emirati conception of the good can be found in its pioneering "second wave" initiative. In 2016, the UAE established a Ministry of Happiness within the federal government, designed to promote a National Programme for Happiness and Positivity (a National Charter for Happiness)

(UAE 2019a). The UAE Declaration of Happiness and Positivity states that "Happiness is the ultimate goal of the UAE government" (UAE 2018, p. 6). The programme is structured around six domains: the development of "World class Healthcare, a Competitive Knowledge Economy, a Safe Public and Fair Judiciary, a First rate Education System, Sustainable Environment and Infrastructure, and a Cohesive Society and Preserved Identity" (UAE 2019b). These domains overlap with the spheres of well-being set out in the Cairo Declaration of Human Rights in Islam, as well as other international frameworks such as the Sustainable Development Goals. As in other places, the importance of "the UAE's unique culture, heritage and traditions" (UAE 2019b) in the individual and collective identities of citizens, is highlighted as a crucial part of the social setting of well-being. The UAE's conception of happiness as "a holistic approach to development, wellbeing and prosperity" (UAE 2018, p. 6) aligns with the Sustainable Development Goals, and with theoretical approaches such as Communitarianism, which conceive of the good life in holistic terms. Overall then, the political principles of the good life found in Qatar's constitution and the UAE's second wave initiative demonstrate that these Middle Eastern countries, which are often set in opposition to the "West" and perceived to have very different value systems, in fact share fundamental value priorities with other countries of the global north and south.

7.3 Mass Priorities in Asia

So far we have discussed philosophical and political conceptions of the good in different parts of Asia. Next we turn to what citizens believe to be most important in life. Table 7.1 shows data from the World Values Survey for a selection of countries in East, South, West, and Central Asia. The values are listed in order of importance for each country.

Table 7.1 shows that, across this diverse range of countries and cultures, as in other regions, a clear margin of priority is given to family relationships. There is wide variation in the importance given to other values. For example, the importance of religion varies starkly, most obviously in the proportions of the populations rating it as "Very important" in China (2.6%) and Iraq (84.7%). A range of historical and political factors contribute to such a large difference in this and other cases. But in the midst of very different histories, cultures and political contexts, the top priority of family ties is a constant theme.

Table 7.1 Value priorities in a selection of Asian countries (% "Very important")

Azerbaijan		*China*		*India*		*Iraq*		*Japan*		*Thailand*	
Family	93.8	Family	85.7	Family	94.9	Family	92.9	Family	90.8	Family	88.6
Work	67.4	Friends	46.6	Work	77.3	Religion	84.7	Work	52.1	Work	66.6
Friends	40.7	Work	38.1	Religion	67.1	Work	66.0	Friends	45.0	Religion	56.6
Religion	35.9	Leisure	21.2	Friends	44.9	Friends	47.8	Leisure	42.3	Friends	32.3
Leisure	21.4	Politics	10.4	Leisure	34.9	Leisure	16.8	Politics	23.5	Politics	32.0
Politics	7.7	Religion	2.6	Politics	17.0	Politics	12.2	Religion	5.4	Leisure	26.4

Source WVS6 (Ingelehart et al. 2014)

7.4 Chapter Summary

The term "Asia" refers to a huge geographical region and a hugely diverse range of countries, with very different cultures and ways of life. However, common threads emerge from the various philosophical traditions and modern socio-political settings. Communitarian values are widespread: the importance of community relationships in the good life is expressed in multiple ways. In the Confucian and Hindu traditions, social relationships are a necessary condition of well-being, since it is through social relationships that virtue is learnt and put into practice. The focus of these traditions on the everyday practicalities of the good life also links to the Communitarian claim that the good and its constituents—Justice for example—are not merely abstract ideals, but must be understood in relation to the social settings in which people's lives are embedded, including the traditions, customs and norms of those communities.

A feature of a good life that arises repeatedly is Benevolence (care, compassion, kindness and charity). This can be seen as one aspect of good social relationships, and provides a link between these theories and feminist philosophy, particularly the ethics of care (e.g. Kittay and Feder 2003). On the feminist view, persons are interdependent, and personhood and well-being are achieved through interpersonal relationships. These principles are at the heart of traditional and modern conceptions of the good in this region.

Protection of cultural heritage and participation in cultural life are ubiquitous features of the constitutions. This may be interpreted as the good of belonging to a social group with whom one shares identities and ends; this is connected to the value of Integrity. A final theme to emerge across the traditions is relationality of a different kind—namely relations to another, non-human, "higher" dimension of knowledge, meaning or understanding, sometimes achieved through religious and spiritual practices. Thoughtfulness (mindfulness) and contemplation are central to the good life. In sum, Social relationships, Cultural participation, and the contemplative life are at the centre of the ethical traditions discussed in this chapter.

References

Ames, R. T., & Rosemont, H. (1998). *The Analects of Confucius: A Philosophical Translation*. New York: Ballantine Books.

Aristotle. (1976). *Nicomachean Ethics* (J. A. K. Thomson, Trans.). London: Penguin Classics.

Chan, J. (2009). Sustainability: A Daoist perspective. In K.-T. Ip (Ed.), *Environmental Ethics: Intercultural Perspectives* (pp. 133–143). Amsterdam: Editions Rodopi B.V.

Cleary, T. (1992). Introduction. In T. Cleary (Trans.), *The Essential Confucius* (pp. 1–11). New York: HarperCollins.

Dahlsgaard, K., Peterson, C., & Seligman, M. E. (2005). Shared virtue: The convergence of valued human strengths across culture and history. *Review of General Psychology, 9*(3), 203–213.

Haberman, D. L. (1998a). Confucianism: The way of the sages. In L. Stevenson & D. L. Haberman (Eds.), *Ten Theories of Human Nature*. New York: Oxford University Press.

Haberman, D. L. (1998b). Upanishadic Hinduism: Quest for ultimate knowledge. In L. Stevenson & D. L. Haberman (Eds.), *Ten Theories of Human Nature* (3rd ed., pp. 45–67). New York: Oxford University Press.

Hacker, P. (2006). Dharma in Hinduism. *Journal of Indian Philosophy, 34*(5), 479–496.

Hasse, D. N. (2018). Influence of Arabic and Islamic philosophy on the Latin West. In E. N. Zalta (Ed.), *The Stanford Encyclopedia of Philosophy* (Winter 2018 ed.). https://plato.stanford.edu/archives/win2018/entries/arabic-islamic-influence/.

Huang, C. (Ed.). (1997). *The analects of Confucius*. Oxford University Press on Demand.

Inglehart, R., Haerpfer, C., Moreno, A., Welzel, C., Kizilova, K., Diez-Medrano, J., et al. (Eds.). (2014). *World Values Survey: Round Six—Country-Pooled Datafile Version*. www.worldvaluessurvey.org/WVSDocumentationWV6.jsp. Madrid: JD Systems Institute.

Kittay, E. F., & Feder, E. K. (2003). *The Subject of Care: Feminist Perspectives on Dependency*. Lanham, MD: Rowman & Littlefield.

Nelson, E. S. (2009). Responding with Dao: Early Daoist ethics and the environment. *Philosophy East and West, 59*(3), 294–316.

UAE. (2018). Nation declaration of happiness and positivity. In *A Guide to Happiness and Wellbeing in the Workplace* (p. 6). https://www.hw.gov.ae/en/download/a-guide-to-happiness-and-wellbeing-program-in-the-workplace-1. Accessed 15 April 2019.

UAE. (2019a). *National Programme for Happiness and Positivity*. https://government.ae/en/about-the-uae/the-uae-government/government-of-future/happiness. Accessed 15 April 2019.

UAE. (2019b). *National Agenda 2021*. https://www.vision2021.ae/en/national-agenda-2021. Accessed 15 April 2019.

Ura, K., Alkire, S., Zangmo, T., & Wangdi, K. (2012). *A Short Guide to Gross National Happiness Index*. Thimphu: The Centre for Bhutan Studies.

Wong, D. (2018). Chinese ethics. In E. N. Zalta (Ed.), *The Stanford Encyclopedia of Philosophy* (Fall 2018 ed.). https://plato.stanford.edu/archives/fall2018/entries/ethics-chinese/. Accessed February 2019.

Yao, H. C., & Yao, X. (2000). *An introduction to Confucianism*. Cambridge University Press.

Yu, J. (2007). *The Ethics of Confucius and Aristotle: Mirrors of Virtue*. New York: Routledge.

CHAPTER 8

Well-being in Africa

Abstract This chapter presents evidence relating to political conceptions of well-being in Africa. First, the southern African philosophy of *Ubuntu* is discussed, and areas of overlap with other ethical frameworks are explored. Next, the national constitutions of countries in North, East, West and Southern Africa are examined, with the aim of identifying the central principles of the political settings of well-being in these countries. Findings from the World Values Survey give a broad view of mass priorities across the region. The analysis shows numerous commonalities, including Material living standards, Health, Education, Work, Community and Family, Political and Cultural Participation, and access to a healthy Natural Environment as constituents of a good life. Also apparent across the national constitutions is the aim of maintaining and developing each country's national identity, including through the blending of traditional and modern customs and values. This can be interpreted as a recognition of the importance of shared histories, traditions and cultures, in political and ethical reasoning at the national, community and individual levels. *Belonging* is a crucial aspect of the good life. To summarise, the dominant commonality to emerge at each of the philosophical, political and civilian levels is the value of harmonious social relationships.

Keywords Well-being · Africa · *Ubuntu* · Values

A. Austin, *A Universal Declaration of Human Well-being*,
Wellbeing in Politics and Policy,
https://doi.org/10.1007/978-3-030-27107-7_8

This chapter presents evidence from Africa. First, the southern African philosophy of *Ubuntu* is discussed, and areas of overlap with other ethical frameworks are explored. Next, the national constitutions of a selection of countries from North, East, West and Southern Africa are examined in order to identify the central principles of political conceptions of the good. Findings from the World Values Survey for Ghana, Morocco, Rwanda, South Africa and Zimbabwe give a broad view of mass priorities across the region.

8.1 Ubuntu: A Philosophy of the Good Life

The *Ubuntu* philosophy found across sub-Saharan Africa can be summarised roughly as meaning "I am because we are" (Van Norren 2014, p. 256). While the term *Ubuntu* encompasses a family of views with different names and nuances in different languages and traditions, all of these views coalesce around a particular worldview, on which human beings are one part of an interconnected system of being, constituted by other humans, all other living things, the ecological habitat and the spiritual world (Gade 2012). In relation to human life, Ngcoya (2009, p. 1) describes how *Ubuntu* is about "the importance of community, solidarity, caring, and sharing. This worldview advocates a profound sense of interdependence and emphasizes that our true human potential can only be realized in partnership with others." *Ubuntu* is similar in these respects to the family of views known as *Buen Vivir* in Latin America (Chapter 6), to the Hindu concept of *Brahman* and the Chinese conception of *Dao* (Chapter 7).

Because it is such a radically different worldview to those found in the English-speaking world, the translation and interpretation of *Ubuntu* is fraught with difficulty and the potential for misuse (Maluleke 1999). However, it is safe to say that, as a social ethic of well-being, there are links between *Ubuntu* and Aristotelian ethics, Communitarianism and Feminist ethics.

There are at least two clear links between *Ubuntu* and Aristotle's ethics. First, for Aristotle, well-being is a matter of a person being and doing well in the social world. The fundamental sociality of well-being is a shared feature of Aristotelian ethics and *Ubuntu*. Second is the connection at the level of human virtues. Aristotle argued that flourishing as a human being means possessing, and acting in accordance with, a set of qualities and attributes ("virtues"). In an investigation of the many meanings of *Ubuntu*, Gade (2012) identified two different ways of understanding the concept. One way is as a general worldview—an ontology of what it is to be human as part of a holistic, interconnected system. The other way is as "a moral quality of a person." For example, Desmond Tutu characterised a person who possesses *Ubuntu* as "generous, hospitable, friendly, caring and compassionate" (Tutu 1999, cited in Gade 2012). This is not dissimilar to the list of virtues set out by Aristotle and other ancient philosophers.

Connections to communitarian and feminist ethics (see Chapter 2) are also apparent in *Ubuntu*. First, communitarianism and *Ubuntu* share an emphasis on the importance of community as (1) a fact of human life and (2) a necessary part of a *good* human life, an indispensable factor in ethical reasoning about the good life and the good society. The *Ubuntu* conception of the person as an inherently social being, defined not by her independence but by her interdependence and caring relationships with others, is also found in feminist ethics.

In some countries (e.g. South Africa), *Ubuntu* has explicitly informed political conceptions of the good; however, as in Latin America, the translation of these traditional principles into modern public policy is open to question and criticism (e.g. Qobo and Nyathi 2016). The next section examines political conceptions of the good in different parts of the continent.

8.2 Constitutional Settings of Well-being

In this section the constitutions of countries across West Africa (Ghana), East Africa (Rwanda), Southern Africa (Zimbabwe) and North Africa (Morocco) are examined, plus the African Charter on Human and Peoples' Rights. The objective is to identify the main principles and values of the political settings of well-being in these different places.

8.2.1 Ghana (1992, Rev. 1996)

The preamble of the constitution of Ghana begins with a statement of "our natural and inalienable right to establish a framework of government which shall secure for ourselves and posterity the blessings of liberty, equality of opportunity and prosperity." The preamble goes on to declare a "commitment to Freedom, Justice and Accountability," and the "protection and preservation of Fundamental Human Rights and Freedoms, Unity and Stability for our nation." These are the guiding principles of the Ghanaian political setting of well-being.

In addition to a section on Fundamental Human Rights and Freedoms based on the International Bill of Rights, the constitution includes sections on the protection of Lands and Natural Resources (Chapter 21), and of the traditional institution of Chieftaincy (Chapter 22). Further on, a section on Political Objectives (Chapter 35) declares that a central aim of the State is "to seek the well-being of all her citizens" through "respect for fundamental human rights and freedoms and the dignity of the human person" (35.2–4). Among the State's Economic Objectives (Chapter 36) are the management of the national economy "in such manner as to maximize the rate of economic development, freedom and happiness of every person in Ghana and to provide adequate means of livelihood and suitable employment and public assistance to the needy" (36.1). Chapter 37 on Social Objectives reiterates the "ideals and principles of freedom, equality, justice, probity and accountability" (37.1), and sets out policy objectives in relation to participation in development processes (37.2.a), and in sport, "as a means of fostering national integration, health and self-discipline." Chapter 38 is devoted to Educational Objectives, and Chapter 39 to Cultural Objectives, including the ambition to "encourage the integration of appropriate customary values into the fabric of national life" (39.1) and to foster pride in Ghanaian culture (39.4). Finally, a number of duties of Ghanaian citizens are set out, including the duty to "live in harmony with others" (41.c) and to "contribute to the well-being of the community where that citizen lives" (41.g).

While Ghana's constitution is strongly guided by international human rights instruments, within this general framework it emphasises particular areas of life that are particularly important on the Ghanaian political conception of the good. The main body of the constitution emphasises Social relationships, Health, Work and livelihood, Living standards, Cultural participation and the economy, political culture and natural environment. Well-being and Freedom are conceptualised as rights of every person, balanced with duties around community and living in harmony with others. It is notable that participation in sport is guaranteed state support as an effective way of nurturing social relations. The ambition to combine the "appropriate" values of tradition and modernity into a distinctive Ghanaian culture, of which citizens can be proud, is also notable. In sum, the constitution of Ghana sets out a vision of a political-economic-social-cultural setting in which individual well-being is achieved within strong communities, drawing on the best parts of local traditions and modern ways of life.

8.2.2 *Morocco (2011)*

The preamble of Morocco's constitution (2011) states a number of principles, including "participation, pluralism, good governance," and "a society of solidarity where all enjoy security, liberty, equality of opportunities, of respect for their dignity and for social justice." Special mention is made of religion: "The pre-eminence accorded to the Muslim religion in the national reference is consistent with the attachment of the Moroccan people to the values of openness, of moderation, of tolerance and of dialog for mutual understanding between all the cultures and the civilizations of the world." In the same vein, the constitution declares that the state is founded on the "values and immutable principles" of "the Rights of Man such as they are universally recognized," and commits to "deepen the bonds of togetherness with the Arab and Islamist Ummah" [the global community of those who share the beliefs and values of Islam].

To promote sustainable human development, the constitution instates a set of public institutions in support of Education (Art.168), the Family and childhood (Art.169), and Youth and Associative life (Art.170). Also included are equal rights to healthcare, social protection, education, decent housing, work, access to public services according to need, and access to water and to a healthy environment (Art.31)

As in other countries, Morocco's constitution is founded in the international treaties and conventions to which it is a signatory, including the Cairo Declaration of Human Rights in Islam. Within this international framework, the values of Participation, Security and Liberty are emphasised. Health, Education, and decent Housing and Work are singled out for constitutional guarantee. Religion is a particularly important part of the Moroccan conception of the good, and is seen as the social glue that binds Moroccan society together. The identification with the Ummah is in some respects similar to other instances of identification with larger systems of meaning and value, such as the "communities of value" found in traditional models of *Buen Vivir* in Latin America (Chapter 6).

8.2.3 *Rwanda (2003, Rev. 2015)*

The preamble of the constitution of Rwanda begins with a statement in honour of "our valiant ancestors…and the heroes who struggled for security, justice, freedom and the restoration of our national tranquillity, dignity and pride." It declares the State's commitment to "upholding our values based on family, morality and patriotism" and working for the "common interest" through "respect for human rights, freedom and the principle of equality." A "fundamental principle" of the state is to "promote social welfare" (Art.10.5), and to develop "home-grown solutions": "In order to build the nation, promote national culture and restore dignity, Rwandans, based on their values, initiate home-grown mechanisms to deal with matters that concern them" (Art.11). As in other places, the value of shared identities and goals looms large in the Rwandan constitution.

In addition to the social, economic, political and civil rights of the International Bill of Human Rights, Chapter V contains a set of duties, including responsibilities to "take part in activities aimed at good health" (Art.45); to "maintain good relations with others" (Art.46); to "protect, safeguard and promote the environment" (Art.53); and to "safeguard and promote national values based on cultural traditions and practices so long as they do not conflict with human rights, public order and good morals...[and] to preserve the national cultural heritage" (Art.47). A further central duty relates to development: "All Rwandans have the duty to participate in the development of the country through their dedication to work, safeguarding peace, democracy, equality and social justice as well as to participate in the defence of their country" (Art.48).

The Rwandan constitution must be interpreted in light of the country's history, including colonialism and the horrors of the 1994 genocide, and as the subject of extensive international development support. It outlines a vision of a society based on social and political institutions aligned with international law, while also maintaining the "national cultural heritage" and building and re-building national identity. From among the basic rights, Health, Social relationships, Environmental protection and Work receive special attention. Overall, the constitution conveys a message that human development and well-being are very much a collective effort, and the institutions of the state and society are designed to promote this collective endeavour.

8.2.4 Zimbabwe (2013, Rev. 2017)

The Preamble of the Zimbabwean constitution sets out a comprehensive set of Zimbabwean values and political goals. These include "freedom, justice and equality"; "Honouring our forebears"; "Celebrating the vibrancy of our traditions and culture"; and "Acknowledging the supremacy of Almighty God, in whose hands our future lies." These value and principles are the foundation of "a united, just and prosperous nation, founded on values of transparency, equality, freedom, fairness, honesty and the dignity of hard work."

Further to this, Chapter 1 affirms the State's "Founding values and principles," which include respect for "fundamental human rights and freedoms" (Art.3.1c) and for "the nation's diverse cultural, religious and traditional values" (Art.3.1d). Cultural life receives further attention, with the provision that "The State and all institutions and agencies of government at every level, and all Zimbabwean citizens, must endeavour to preserve and protect Zimbabwe's heritage...[including] cultural values and practices which enhance the dignity, well-being and equality of Zimbabweans [and] due respect for the dignity of traditional institutions" (Art.16).

The social, economic, political and civil rights of the IBHR are included (Part 2), with the addition of a separate article on Environmental Rights, including the right of every person to a healthy environment, and the ecologically sustainable development of natural resources for economic and social development (Art.73).

Overall, and similarly to the other constitutions examined in this section, the Zimbabwean constitution sets out a vision of society that is strongly guided by international instruments such as the IBHR. Within this framework of human rights, progress and well-being occur in a social-political context that includes the diversity of customs and traditions of the region, in combination with the policies and practices of modern development initiatives.

8.2.5 The African Charter on Human and Peoples' Rights

The African Charter on Human and Peoples' Rights is an initiative of the intergovernmental organisation, the African Union. Articles 1–18 of the Charter contain the social, economic, cultural, political and civil rights of individuals, as they are found in the International Bill of Rights. This part of the Charter also guarantees protection for "traditional values recognized by the community" (e.g. Art.17.3). Articles 19–25 list a set of rights of peoples, that is, of collectivities. The recognition of groups as rights-bearers can be seen in the light of the histories of modern African states, many of which have seen violence of various kinds against specific ethnic and racial groups. Overall, then, the Charter aligns with the aim expressed in national constitutions of promoting human rights within a context informed by those aspects of national identity deemed to be most important.

To summarise the discussion of political conceptions of the good, the constitutions discussed here all take a rights-based approach to defining the broad parameters of the political setting of well-being. Individual and collective rights are expected to be fulfilled within a communitarian setting: harmonious social relationships are a core value, and there are many references to living and working together for the common good. The religious and spiritual life figures more prominently than in other regions. The goal of blending modern and traditional values and practices is of central importance in every case.

8.3 Mass Priorities in Africa

The discussion so far has focused on philosophical and political conceptions of the good. We now turn to the mass priorities of civilian populations. Table 8.1 shows data from the World Values Survey for a selection of African countries from North, East, West and Southern Africa. The values are listed in order of importance for each country.

The results show that, in countries across the African continent, as is the case in all of the other regions under consideration, family relationships are most likely to be seen as "Very important" (although similar proportions in Ghana and Morocco also prioritise work and religion respectively). Beyond the top priority accorded to family relationships, there is considerable variation in the mass priorities of these countries. The shared prioritisation of family relationships is consistent with the constitutions examined above, all of which emphasise the value of communality, and guarantee state protection for different forms of social relationships.

8.4 Chapter Summary

The continent (and concept) of Africa is hugely diverse, in terms of geography, history, tradition, language and culture. As such, generalisations can be made only at the highest level. This chapter has shown that, in line with international law, the constitutions of the African countries considered here are rights-based. All include constitutional guarantees of the goods of Resources adequate to meet basic needs, Health, Education, Work, Community and Family, Political and Cultural Participation, and access to a healthy Natural Environment. At the same time as adhering to international agreements, apparent across these national constitutions is the aim of maintaining and developing each country's national identity, including through

Table 8.1 Value priorities in a selection of African countries (% "Very important")

Ghana		*Morocco*		*Rwanda*		*South Africa*		*Zimbabwe*	
Family	95.9	Family	90.7	Family	91.7	Family	92.5	Family	97.3
Work	94.8	Religion	88.9	Friends	72.1	Work	57.5	Work	85.4
Religion	91.1	Work	82.5	Work	70.5	Religion	55.8	Religion	83.5
Leisure time	51.9	Friends	35.8	Religion	40.3	Friends	44.7	Leisure time	38.7
Friends	45.7	Leisure time	16.9	Leisure time	31.4	Leisure time	36.1	Friends	37.8
Politics	22.5	Politics	6.2	Politics	21.1	Politics	21.4	Politics	20.7

Source WVS 6 (Inglehart et al. 2014)

the promotion and protection of the best parts of culturally-specific traditions and values. This represents a recognition of the importance of the rich particularities of history, tradition and culture, in political and ethical reasoning at the national, community and individual levels. Emerging from these diverse expressions of well-being, however, the common theme of the value of harmonious social relationships emerges at each of the philosophical, political and civilian levels.

References

Gade, C. B. (2012). What is Ubuntu? Different interpretations among South Africans of African descent. *South African Journal of Philosophy, 31*(3), 484–503.

Inglehart, R., Haerpfer, C., Moreno, A., Welzel, C., Kizilova, K., Diez-Medrano, J., et al. (Eds.). (2014). *World Values Survey: Round Six—Country-Pooled Datafile Version*. www.worldvaluessurvey.org/WVSDocumentationWV6.jsp. Madrid: JD Systems Institute.

Maluleke, T. (1999). The misuse of '*Ubuntu*'. *Challenge, 53,* 12–13.

Ngcoya, M. (2009). *Ubuntu: Globalization, Accommodation, and Contestation in South Africa*. Washington, DC: American University.

Qobo, M., & Nyathi, N. (2016). Ubuntu, public policy ethics and tensions in South Africa's foreign policy. *South African Journal of International Affairs, 23*(4), 421–436.

Van Norren, D. E. (2014). The nexus between Ubuntu and Global Public Goods: Its relevance for the post 2015 development Agenda. *Development Studies Research: An Open Access Journal, 1*(1), 255–266.

PART II

Summary of Part II: Well-being in Practice

Part II has reviewed the political and legal instruments that form the political settings of well-being across the world. It also examined "second wave" national initiatives, and findings from the World Values Survey regarding the mass priorities of populations.

The preceding chapters have shown that human rights are at the core of national constitutions, with the rights drawn from international agreements including both the International Bill of Human Rights, and the Cairo Declaration of Human Rights in Islam. While the national constitutions share their basis in human rights, the nuances of the relevant sections, including omissions, emphases and wordings, show that the basic rights are prioritised and manifested differently in different places.

The constitutions display various shades of the theories discussed in Part I: The values associated with Political Liberalism (individual freedom) and Communitarianism (social embeddedness) are found to different extents in different places, in various combinations, and moderated by different considerations according to national histories and priorities. While there is no guarantee that constitutional principles will be successfully translated into effective policy, the constitutions nevertheless set out the values and ideals that, in theory at least, set the parameters of the political settings of well-being.

At the national and regional levels, responses to the call to go "Beyond GDP" take many forms. The second wave "Beyond GDP" initiatives are found mainly in the higher income OECD countries, and have been guided by the pioneering OECD programme. However, these domains of value are not unique to OECD countries: the example of Bhutan confirms this. The OECD domains are also emphasised in many non-OECD countries; for example, Material living standards, Health, Education, Work, Community and family, Political participation, Cultural participation and the Natural environment are emphasised in the Ghanaian and Indian constitutions.

Finally, the findings from the World Values Survey provide a very clear message: in every country of every region considered, Family was the most important aspect of a good life. The WVS can give only a very broad view of mass priorities; it shows only what is important among the six values on the pre-defined list. However, the values analysed here span different spheres of life, and the findings are sufficient to show a clear pattern. Close social relationships are at the heart of well-being.

The consensus spheres of value emerging from Part II can be summarised as follows:

- Social relationships (family, community, formal social institutions)
- Material security (resources to meet the physical needs of decent nutrition, shelter, clothing, etc.)
- Health (physical and psychological)
- Work (including work-life balance)
- Leisure
- Education
- Natural environment (access and concern for)
- Political participation
- Cultural participation
- Integrity (Harmony between practical reasoning and practical action).

Part III brings together the different strands of analysis, to show that universals of human well-being can be distilled from wide-ranging cultural diversity.

PART III

Well-being: A Reflective Equilibrium

Parts I and II have set out evidence about well-being in theory, and well-being in practice. Part III seeks equilibrium between these different sources of knowledge, in order to identify common ground among conceptions of the good across the world.

CHAPTER 9

Well-being: A Reflective Equilibrium

Abstract The question of what it means to live well has been debated in the public forum for millennia, and continues to occupy a central place in politics and policy. The starting hypothesis of this study was that, if people across the world, from different cultures, languages and worldviews, share common values, and if these overlap with philosophical theories of well-being, then this is evidence that there are good reasons and reason to value those things. This chapter brings together the different strands of analysis to identify common ground between theoretical and practical accounts of well-being. The final analysis shows that good social relationships are a necessary condition of all the other constituents of a good life. Happiness and freedom require other people, and good health, work, education and leisure are grounded in meaningful, mutually respectful social connections. Belonging—the sharing of identities, interests and ends with others—grounds well-being. For politics and policy, focusing on Sociality would reap dividends: Good social relationships are a catalyst of overall well-being. The biggest lesson for politics and policy is that the journey Beyond GDP should be directed towards building a sound infrastructure of sociality to underpin well-being.

Keywords Values · Well-being · Sociality · Beyond GDP

A. Austin, *A Universal Declaration of Human Well-being*,
Wellbeing in Politics and Policy,
https://doi.org/10.1007/978-3-030-27107-7_9

The question of what it means to live well is arguably the most important human question of all. It has been debated in the public forum for millennia, and continues to occupy a central place in politics and policy. Given the common features of human existence, including our shared physical embodiment and shared sociality, it would be surprising if there were no common ground in what it means to live well. While there are obvious universals of human life, including the basic needs of physical survival such as food and shelter, this study has been concerned with the universals not just of human life, but of a *good* human life. My starting hypothesis was that there is a universal core of human well-being, and that the elements of this universal core are discoverable. The objective was to find a balance between diverse theoretical and practical sources of information about well-being, to arrive at a stable account of well-being that would satisfy the demands of both philosophy and practical politics and policy, each as a check and balance on the other.

The analysis employed a central insight of Sen's Capability Approach: that well-being is a question of the freedoms and opportunities people have to live "the lives they value – and have reason to value" (Sen 1999). Identifying what people actually value can provide evidence about what there is reason to value. If people across the world, from different cultures, with different languages and worldviews, share common values, and if these overlap with philosophical theories of well-being, then this is evidence that there are good reasons and reason to value those things. This chapter brings together the different strands of analysis, to identify common ground between theoretical and practical accounts of well-being.

9.1 Themes from Theory

A review of foundational ethical theories gave rise to an initial set of basic values of a good human life: Happiness (from Hedonism); Freedom (from Liberalism); and Sociality (from Aristotelian ethics). However, questions remained. What causes and constitutes happiness? What, more specifically, do we want freedom for: Freedom to what? What does the basic fact of our sociality enable us to do, have and be?

Answers to these questions, developed through philosophical methods, added detail and extended the initial set of candidate universals:

- Sociality (Harmonious, mutually respectful social relationships, including family, friendship, community and the formal institutions of sociality)
- Pleasure (Subjective well-being, happiness, emotional well-being)
- Freedom (Liberties and rights)
- Education
- Meaningful work
- Leisure (Rest, recreation, play)
- Material security
- Health (Physical and mental, the latter including self-respect)
- Connection with the natural environment
- Aesthetic experience
- Integrity (Harmony between practical reasoning and practical action).

Each of these goods are included in some way in multiple theoretical accounts of well-being. For example, meaningful Work and Leisure, and Education and the development of the mind, are found across time and tradition. Particularly notable is the ubiquity of sociality. The importance of good and mutually respectful social relationships is emphasised in ancient Chinese, ancient Indian, and ancient Greek philosophy, and in modern political theory, from Rawls' Kantian-inspired Political liberalism to Aristotelian-inspired accounts of the good life. This is consistent with the "social conception of the person" found in Aristotelian and feminist ethics. The human person is a social animal, dependent on and defined by her social relationships. Children are "called into personhood" (Lindemann 2016) by their families and communities, and all persons live their lives in social settings. These settings are a necessary part of practical reasoning and practical action, and therefore Integrity. Human life is founded in sociality, and therefore so is a *good* human life.

To summarise, the list above represents the common ground among theoretical accounts of well-being, and from these, good social relationships are identified as having special importance, as both a good in themselves, and as a condition of the other constituents of well-being.

Identifying this common ground across theories from very different traditions is the first step in balancing theoretical conceptions, principles and considered judgements with their practical counterparts, into a reflective equilibrium on well-being.

9.2 Themes from Practice

Turning to practice, a number of themes emerged from the three strands of analysis: first, the political settings of well-being defined by international law and national constitutions; second, "Beyond GDP" national well-being programmes; and third, the World Values Survey.

9.2.1 The Constitutional Settings of Well-being

Part II showed that the idea of well-being in politics and policy in the modern era has been grounded in a rights-based conception of the good; national constitutions and international legal instruments demonstrate this. The central role of rights in defining the political settings of well-being across the world can be explained by the influence, in global governance, of the liberal democracies of the global North. However, within the context of universal rights, there is also universal emphasis on particularities—on the expression of distinctive national identities, histories and cultural heritage, and the rights and capabilities of citizens to participate in this, as both a personal and shared good. This suggests a conception of well-being in which individual and collective self-respect is grounded in belonging to a particular tradition and culture. This observation resonates with the communitarian claim that the shared ends, identities, values and interests that define communities are a necessary part of human life, and reasoning about the good cannot be conducted in isolation from these social settings. As in theoretical accounts, Sociality is fundamental.

The value of Integrity is implicated here. Personal well-being happens in a setting. This setting is partly defined by social history and cultural heritage. Histories and heritages are the basis of ongoing narratives and shared identities, and are a rich resource that can be drawn upon by groups and individuals in public deliberation and practical reasoning. Histories, heritage and identities are always contestable, and so protecting citizens' capabilities to participate in ongoing cultural narratives is an important political goal, and an important means of guarding against the manipulation of such narratives for harmful ends (e.g. through propaganda or suppression of dissent). Integrity at the personal level (harmony between practical reasoning and practical action) is grounded in sociality, and both aspects of Integrity (practical reasoning and practical action) involve shared ends, identities and interests.

In addition to Freedom, Community and Integrity, the constitutions put varying degrees of emphasis on the substantive goods of Education, Health and health care, Family and social relationships (often expressed in terms of "solidarity"), Material living standards, Work, Natural environment, Justice and security, Political participation and Cultural participation. These often appear in the sections on rights and duties, and are derived from the fundamental rights of the IBHR, but at the same time are worded or emphasised in ways that reflect national priorities. An example of this is the special emphasis in the constitution of India (2016) on the right to work (Art.41); on securing "just and humane conditions of work" (Art.42); and a living wage that enables "a decent standard of life…" (Art.43). These particularly detailed constitutional guarantees of decent work are designed to promote the welfare of historically disadvantaged groups, in support of the "Abolition of Untouchability" (Art.17). The particularities in the expression and prioritisation of rights across different national constitutions is an example of the multiple realizability thesis (see Chapter 1), whereby common ground underlies surface diversity.

While there is no guarantee that constitutional principles will be successfully put into practice, the constitutions nevertheless represent the principles of ideal political settings of well-being, and the conceptions of the good that these settings are designed to support.

9.2.2 "Beyond GDP" Initiatives

Many of the conditions and constituents of well-being found in constitutions also appear in "second wave" Beyond GDP initiatives. These initiatives, found mostly in the higher income countries, converged on the following domains:

- Health (physical and mental)
- Material security (resources to meet the physical needs of decent nutrition, housing, clothing, etc.)
- Social relationships (family, friends, community, formal social institutions)
- Political and civic participation
- Cultural participation
- Subjective well-being (happiness, life-satisfaction, self-respect)
- Work (including work-life balance)
- Rest and leisure

- Natural environment (engagement with the natural world)
- Economy
- Education
- Good governance
- Safety and security.

The second wave initiatives and constitutions alike include domains relating to both individual level and national-level well-being. Health, Happiness and so on apply at the individual level, while Economy and Good governance are state-level factors. For example, the "Economy" domain found in Beyond GDP initiatives relates to the economic setting of well-being, and is also found in constitutional guarantees such as the Ghanaian commitment to manage the national economy "in such manner as to maximize the rate of economic development, freedom and happiness of every person in Ghana" (Art.36.1). This is consistent with the idea that individual well-being occurs within a social-political-economic setting, and depends on that setting.

9.2.3 *The World Values Survey*

Findings from the World Values Survey give a broad view of mass priorities in different regions. While the findings must be interpreted within the constraints of the data, the results demonstrate one very clear pattern: Across the vast range of languages, cultures, histories, political contexts, and stages of development, of utmost importance in people's lives are family relationships. Close social relationships are at the heart of well-being. This is yet another example of the special place of social relationships in human being, and human well-being.

9.3 Overlapping Values

As well as overlapping with one another, the spheres of value that emerged from the review of well-being in Practice also overlap with many of the themes that emerged from the theories of well-being reviewed in Part I. Comparing the spheres of value that emerged from the theories and practices of well-being results in the following list of goods that are valued consistently in theoretical conceptions of well-being, in political and policy practice, and in the mass priorities of national populations:

- Sociality (Harmonious, mutually respectful social relationships, including family, friendship, community, and the formal institutions of sociality)
- Material security (resources to meet the physical needs of decent nutrition, housing, clothing, etc.)
- Safety and security
- Subjective well-being (pleasure, happiness, life-satisfaction, emotional well-being, self-respect)
- Health (physical and mental)
- Freedom (self-determination)
- Meaningful work
- Rest and Leisure
- Education
- Political participation
- Cultural participation
- Natural environment (engagement with the natural world)
- Integrity (Harmony between practical reasoning and practical action).

The majority of these spheres of value are uncontroversial. Those relating to the economic, social and environmental resources needed for life and health are universally found in politics and policy, including regimes underpinned by the International Bill of Human Rights and the Cairo Declaration of Human Rights in Islam. These spheres are found across second wave Beyond GDP initiatives, and are also explicitly or implicitly included in the theoretical accounts of the good life considered in Part I. For example, Aristotle discusses the importance of health (e.g. NE 1140a25–26) and material resources (e.g. NE 1096a22) in being able to live a good human life. Similarly, for Rawls, Health and Wealth are "natural" and "social" primary goods respectively (Rawls 1972, p. 62).

Meaningful work and leisure time are uncontroversial. Subjective well-being might be seen as a constituent or a result of a good life, but either way, all else being equal, theory and practice agree that a life of happiness is better than a life of subjective misery. We have seen that cultural and political participation are a crucial part of a good life, particularly because they enable a person to participate in the development of shared identities, ends and interests that provide resources for practical reasoning.

Two spheres deserve special attention: Social relationships and Integrity. Martha Nussbaum (2000) singled out "Affiliation" (social relationships) and "Practical reason" as particularly important in her list of capabilities, because they "organize and suffuse all the others" (p. 82). The present study provides fresh evidence in support of Nussbaum's view, using a different set of sources.

9.3.1 *Social Relationships*

The utmost importance in people's lives of social relationships shines through both the theory and practice of well-being. Sociality has special importance because it is of both intrinsic and instrumental value. That is, it is a constituent of a good human life in its own right, and is also instrumental in the achievement of other goods. This is, first and foremost, simply a descriptive claim. Sociality is a necessary condition of life, and therefore of a good life. Without the care of others, human infants would not survive. From a normative perspective, social isolation is inimical to the well-being of all human beings of all ages. For example, social isolation has negative effects on the health of the isolated individual. An extreme example is the psychological damage caused by solitary confinement in prisons (e.g. Smith 2006). More generally, loneliness, social exclusion and alienation impede well-being. A lonely older person and an alienated youth, for example, are both excluded from opportunities in many other domains, from cultural and political participation to health, education and leisure. Social relationships are what Wolff and de-Shalit (2007) call a "fertile functioning," due to their positive spill-over effects on other domains of well-being.

On some theoretical accounts, a person cannot achieve well-being in isolation from others, because, by definition, living well means living in certain ways towards others. For Aristotle, a good life is defined by virtues such as benevolence. Such other-regarding virtues require others for their exercise. This is not to say that those others are only valuable as means to the person's well-being; rather that a defining feature of being human is having relationships with others, and so being human well involves having good relationships with others.

Social relationships do not only include close family and friends, but extend to a wider circle of community relationships, including place-based social groups of more- or less-known others, and disparate communities defined by shared memories, values or religion. Another aspect of sociality is the formal institutions that enable people to live together: the legal and political institutions of the state. This aspect is described by the primary good of "The social bases of self-respect: the recognition by social institutions that gives citizens a sense of self-worth and the confidence to carry out their plans" (Rawls 2001, pp. 58–59), and is elaborated by national constitutions. Social relationships at all of these levels (personal, community and state) sustain and give meaning to human life. As suggested by Rawls' inclusion of the "social bases of self-respect" as a primary good, individual freedom is fundamentally dependent on sociality.

As we saw above, the fact and value of sociality in human life implies a conception of the person not as a lone individual defined by independence and self-sufficiency, but as an agent who is the product of a multi-layered system of interdependent social relationships, and is embedded in this social setting in such a way that her life and well-being depend on it.

9.3.2 (Relational) Integrity

The second sphere for further discussion is Integrity, defined as harmony between practical reason and practical action. In Sect. 3.2, practical reasoning was defined as the reflective process of developing a conception of the good, and forming plans, projects and commitments based on that conception. "Wide practical reasoning" refers to practical reasoning that draws upon a wide range of resources, including critical engagement with one's social setting in its broadest sense, and theoretical reasoning about the good, for which education provides the tools.

The addition of the prefix "wide" is designed to draw attention to the social embeddedness of every person, and the role of this social embeddedness in practical reasoning. Wide practical reasoning involves recognition of the shared ends, identities and interests that constitute human existence, and incorporation of this into deliberation about the good life. This requires reflective engagement with one's social setting, broadly conceived as the social-political-cultural-material setting of one's life, including the communities of values (see Chapter 6) to which one belongs. The emphasis on national identity and cultural participation found in many constitutions also relates to persons having access to the rich resources of histories and heritages as part of personal practical reasoning. Some conceptions of well-being are explicit in their inclusion of the good of incorporating ancestral wisdom into practical reasoning (e.g. in traditional Latin American and Hindu approaches), and some modern accounts include religion as a means of gaining theoretical knowledge of the good (e.g. Finnis 2011). Reflective engagement with one's setting includes, in some cases, criticism and rebellion against it; this is Aristotle's virtue of "Righteous indignation"

(Nussbaum calls it "Justified anger"). Overall, this demonstrates the social basis of practical reasoning.

The second part of Integrity is practical action in accordance with the conception of the good developed through wide practical reasoning. Being able to act in accordance with one's conception of the good also depends on features of one's social setting, including material, political and cultural features, and social norms and values. Both aspects of Integrity—practical reasoning and practical action—are grounded in sociality. In Sect. 3.2, I proposed the term "Relational Integrity" to describe this good. It is a necessary part of well-being, and cannot be achieved alone.

9.4 Implications for Politics and Policy: An Infrastructure of Sociality

The main finding of this study is that social relationships are not only a central constituent of well-being, but a necessary condition of it. Human beings are social animals, and human well-being is achieved in social settings. In practice, this means that, to support well-being, politics and policy must be grounded in a social conception of the good. This entails a recognition of the interdependence of human beings, and that social relationships are the foundation of life, and therefore of a good life. Politics and policy based on such a conception would focus on building an infrastructure of sociality to support individual and collective well-being. The infrastructure of sociality encompasses close relationships with family and friends, community relationships, and social and political institutions at the local, national and international levels.

Another lesson for politics and policy can be drawn from the ancient traditions that include the natural environment as a basic component of the "setting" of human well-being. Protection of the natural environment, and of people's ability to connect with it, is therefore an important area for policy priority. The Japanese practice of "forest bathing" and "forest therapy" is a good example of how connections to the natural environment can be supported in the modern era (Takayama et al. 2014). Moreover, the concept of environment must be extended to encompass the urban environment in which the majority of the global population lives. Urban planning designed to support sociality and well-being is key.

Politics and policy, in the twentieth century, erroneously inverted the means and ends of human well-being. Prioritising wealth and GDP as the most important end often left people as mere means to achieving a sound economy. Putting this error right requires a shift from an economic conception of the good to a social conception of the good. Economic factors are important, because the material resources required to meet basic needs must be in place for people to develop and follow their own conception of the good. However, enhancing people's capabilities to lead the lives they value and have reason to value requires people-centred politics and policy that makes sociality the end, with economic factors as only a means to this. In addition to tackling inequality in economic wealth, efforts should be concentrated on tackling inequality in what the Bolivians call "social wealth."

For politics and policy, focusing on Sociality would reap dividends: Social relationships have both intrinsic and instrumental value: they are not only a central constituent of well-being in their own right, but are also instrumental in the achievement of other constituents of well-being. Good social relationships have a multiplier effect: they are a catalyst of overall well-being.

9.5 Conclusion: A Universal Declaration of Human Well-being

The aim of this study was to identify the elements of a universal core of well-being, as a tool for people-centred politics and policy. By bringing together theoretical and practical sources of knowledge about well-being, the final analysis shows that there are aspects of human life that are universally valued. The consistency and prevalence of these value-beliefs across time, language, geography, tradition and culture, in theory and in practice, is evidence that there is good reason to value these particular aspects of life. A Universal Declaration of well-being is possible. The central common ground of the Theory and Practice of Well-being is constituted by the values of Good social relationships, Material Security, Safety and Security, Subjective well-being, Health, Freedom (relational autonomy), meaningful Work and Leisure, Education, Political Participation, Cultural Participation, Engagement with the Natural Environment, and Relational Integrity (being able to live in accordance with one's basic convictions about what is most important in life).

The analysis provides support for many existing Beyond GDP initiatives, and for some philosophical conceptions of the good, such as Nussbaum's ten central capabilities. Most importantly, it draws attention to the special importance of Sociality, as a necessary condition of human life, and of a *good* human life. To conclude, the biggest lesson for politics and policy of this study is that the journey Beyond GDP should be directed towards building a sound infrastructure of sociality to underpin and catalyse human well-being.

References

Aristotle. (1976). *The Ethics of Aristotle: The Nicomachean Ethics* (J. A. K. Thomson, Trans.). London: Penguin Classics.

Finnis, J. (2011). *Natural law and natural rights.* Oxford University Press.

Lindemann, H. (2016). *Holding and Letting Go: The Social Practice of Personal Identities.* Oxford: Oxford University Press.

Nussbaum, M. C. (2000). *Women and Human Development: The Capabilities Approach.* Cambridge: Cambridge University Press.

Rawls, J. (1972). *A Theory of Justice.* London: Oxford University Press.

Rawls, J. (2001). *Justice as Fairness: A Restatement.* Cambridge: Harvard University Press.

Sen, A. (1999). *Development as Freedom.* Oxford: Oxford University Press.

Smith, P. S. (2006). The effects of solitary confinement on prison inmates: A brief history and review of the literature. *Crime and Justice, 34*(1), 441–528.

Takayama, N., Korpela, K., Lee, J., Morikawa, T., Tsunetsugu, Y., Park, B. J., et al. (2014). Emotional, restorative and vitalizing effects of forest and urban environments at four sites in Japan. *International Journal of Environmental Research and Public Health, 11*(7), 7207–7230.

Wolff, J., & de-Shalit, A. (2007). *Disadvantage.* Oxford: Oxford University Press on Demand.

Index

A. Austin, *A Universal Declaration of Human Well-being*, Wellbeing in Politics and Policy,
https://doi.org/10.1007/978-3-030-27107-7

Printed by Printforce, the Netherlands